The Pocket Carbohydrate Counter Guide for Diabetes

Simple Nutritional Strategies
to Lower Your Blood Sugar

THE **POCKET**
CARBOHYDRATE
COUNTER
GUIDE
FOR **DIABETES**

**SHELBY
KINNAIRD**

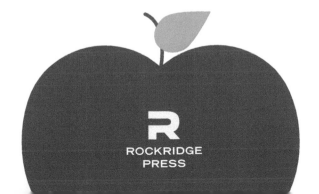

ROCKRIDGE
PRESS

Contents

Introduction

Carbohydrates. The word triggers so many emotions. You may love carbs or hate them. Chances are you sometimes crave them and often spurn them. But if you have diabetes or prediabetes, the critical thing is that you count them. This book will show you how to do that.

Diagnosed with type 2 diabetes in 1999, I've learned to manage it pretty well. Keeping in touch with others via my website, Diabetic Foodie, and my two DiabetesSisters support groups helps me tremendously. One thing I've learned is that everyone needs education and tools to help them stay on track with their diet—especially handling those pesky carbs.

There is no one perfect diet for someone with diabetes or prediabetes. A meal plan one person finds easy to follow may be extremely frustrating for someone else. An eating style that yields in-range blood sugars when you're first diagnosed may produce less than stellar results 15 years later.

The trick is to find tools that help manage your carb intake, regardless of your particular diet or current stage of diabetes. This book is full of those tools.

What you won't find here is an exhaustive list of foods and their carb counts. For that type of nutritional information, there are already plenty of other excellent books, websites, and apps available.

What this book will give you is a brief introduction to carbohydrates and how your body processes them. You'll learn about the different types of carbs and why some are "better" than others. You'll discover how to recognize carbs, especially in foods where they hide. Most important, you'll find out how many carbs you should eat at each meal and learn some clever techniques for staying on track.

HOW TO USE THIS BOOK

It's best to start with the scientific background information in part 1, then continue on to the tools in part 2, and end with the lifestyle tips in part 3.

If you don't have time to read the whole book right now, skip ahead to the "10 Tips" in chapter 11 (page 99). You'll get a nice overview of what the book covers; then later, you can go back and read the "whys" behind the tips in the earlier chapters.

Do you hate math? If so, you'll love the carb-counting alternatives in chapter 5. As someone with two math degrees, however, I must encourage you to eventually tackle chapters 3 and 4. Take a deep breath, give yourself a pep talk, and jump in. Measuring, counting, and tracking can be a huge help in managing your blood sugar, and it's not as hard as you think. Show your middle school math teacher that she was wrong about you!

Are you someone who simply likes to dive in head first—no preparation or advance knowledge required? If this sounds like you, skim the scientific stuff in part 1, and then plunge straight into part 2.

Do you have *type 1 diabetes* or *latent autoimmune diabetes in adults* (LADA)? While the information in this book will help you count carbs and track your blood sugar, I haven't included much to guide you in dosing your insulin beyond the "Insulin Therapy" section in chapter 1 (page 14). For additional assistance, check some of the resources at the end of the book.

DISCLAIMER

I am not a medical professional of any kind: I'm not a doctor, diabetes educator, dietitian, or nutritionist. What I've learned about diabetes has come from reading, talking to people, taking classes, participating in support groups, experimenting with my own diet, attending diabetes conferences, getting involved in the diabetes online community (DOC), and asking medical professionals many, many questions over the years. If I suggest something in this book that contradicts advice given to you by your health care team, please listen to them and not to me.

PART I

The Carbs–Diabetes Connection

When it comes to successfully managing your diabetes—whether you have prediabetes, type 1, type 2, LADA, or gestational diabetes—controlling your carbohydrate intake is crucial. But before you learn how to count carbs, you need to understand the relationship between carbs and diabetes—what happens inside our bodies when we eat the different types of foods. Do carbs affect us in the same way protein does? Will eating as few carbs and as much protein as possible be better for our blood sugar and overall health? What about fats? Should we eat fat or eliminate it from our diet? There are so many questions.

Chapter 1 will take you through the chemistry of how the carbs you eat turn into glucose and how that glucose fuels your body, especially your brain. Don't panic if you hated science in school. I'll explain some basic information that's helpful to understand about your body, and if you can't remember all of the details and technical terms, that's okay. Just focus on the main ideas. You'll also learn about the different types of carbohydrates and why some have less of an effect on your blood sugar than others. At the end of the chapter, I talk about insulin and the different types of *type 2 diabetes* medications your doctor may prescribe.

Chapter 2 will teach you about proteins and fats, what happens when you eat those two types of foods, and how your body processes them differently than carbs. You'll also learn to recognize carbs in foods—including hidden ones—and get information about artificial sweeteners. Finally, I'll point you to some useful carb-counting tools.

CHAPTER ONE

The Science of Blood Sugar

CARBS AND YOUR BODY

Your body needs nutrients to function properly. It requires large quantities of some, known as *macronutrients*, and smaller amounts of others, called *micronutrients*. There are three types of macronutrients: *carbohydrates, proteins*, and *fats*. These do the heavy lifting when it comes to providing energy and keeping your tissues strong. Micronutrients, on the other hand, are the vitamins and minerals your body needs to complete hundreds of jobs every day. Vitamin C, for example, found in citrus fruits, helps heal wounds, while magnesium, found in leafy greens and avocados, helps keep your immune system strong. Eating a wide variety of healthy foods increases the chances that your body receives all the nutrients necessary to function at its maximum potential.

What Are Carbs?

The most important sources of energy for your body, carbohydrates, are naturally found in fruits, vegetables, grains, legumes (e.g., beans), nuts, seeds, and dairy products. You also find carbs in sweet treats, sugary drinks, and processed convenience foods. When you eat carbs, your digestive system turns them into *glucose*, which is used to fuel your cells and your brain. Having access to adequate supplies of glucose is so vital that your body hoards it, keeping an extra supply tucked away in your liver and muscles. This is the reason you can go on functioning even when you haven't eaten recently.

How the Body Processes Carbs

So how do carbs turn into fuel? Everything starts with the body's digestive system, comprising the *gastrointestinal (GI) tract* plus three organs: the liver, pancreas, and gallbladder. The GI tract includes the esophagus, stomach, and intestines (small and large). The food you eat moves through the esophagus, into the stomach, and then into the small intestine. There, the food mixes with digestive juices from the liver and pancreas, and nutrients from the food are absorbed into the bloodstream. Waste products that result from the digestive process end up in the large intestine for storage until they can be eliminated from the body via a bowel movement.

When you eat carbs, your digestive system breaks down the sugars and starches into glucose. The glucose transfers into your bloodstream and raises your blood sugar. *Insulin*, a hormone released by your pancreas (or for some people with diabetes, taken in the form of a shot), unlocks your cells so glucose can enter. When the glucose moves from the bloodstream into the cells, your blood sugar level goes down. Meanwhile, extra glucose is stored in your liver and muscles for future use in the form of *glycogen*.

When the System Doesn't Work

Beta cells in your pancreas produce insulin. People with diabetes have beta cells that are not working properly and, therefore, they don't have enough insulin. Too little insulin for the amount of glucose in the bloodstream means cells won't be fed, so blood sugar will stay elevated, a condition known as *hyperglycemia*. In this case, your kidneys will filter out the excess glucose and, essentially, you'll urinate away the nutrients your body needs to function.

To make matters worse, glucose is "sticky" and can bind to protein. Blood vessels are made of protein, so when glucose hangs around too long, it can attach to blood vessels in your kidneys, eyes, and nerves. This may result in kidney disease, *diabetic retinopathy*, or *diabetic neuropathy*, serious conditions that can lead to kidney failure, blindness, or amputations.

So where does all this information point? If you have diabetes, controlling the amount of carbs you eat, and therefore the amount of glucose in your bloodstream, is essential to maintaining your long-term health.

Carbs and Your Brain

Your brain comprises only about 2 percent of your total body weight, but it uses about 20 percent of your body's resources. Glucose is brain fuel and, as you know, comes from the carbs you eat. Your brain's frontal lobe engages when you actively focus on an idea or make a decision, so it's pretty important to your overall well-being. Since the frontal lobe is quite sensitive to drops in glucose, mental decline is often the first warning sign of a possible nutrient deficiency.

The combination of the sugar, starch, and *fiber* you eat directly affects how well your brain functions. Simple carbs (sugars) cause first a spike and then a dip in glucose levels. This may have negative effects on your attention span and mood. On the other hand, fiber-rich foods like beans and oats release glucose into your bloodstream over a longer period of time; since this provides a more constant supply of fuel for your brain, the effect is a greater ability to concentrate. Sustained brain power results from a regular diet of nutrient-rich foods, including the right kinds of carbs.

TYPES OF CARBOHYDRATES

Carbohydrates may be classified as simple or complex. The more complex carbohydrates are, the longer it takes them to enter your bloodstream as glucose. Taking a closer look:

Simple carbs are sugars found naturally in fruits, vegetables, and dairy products, and are often added to processed foods. Your body can rapidly convert simple carbs into glucose, so eating these causes a quick spike in blood sugar.

Complex carbs are found in whole grains, starchy vegetables, beans, and lentils, and are often a good source of fiber. Your body takes a bit longer to convert complex carbs into glucose; as a result, your blood sugar rises more gradually than it does with simple carbs.

Carbohydrates come in three forms: sugar, starch, and fiber.

Sugar

The simplest form of carbohydrate, sugar is found in sweets, fruits, vegetables, and milk products. As a category, sugars exist either as *monosaccharides* (one sugar molecule) or *disaccharides* (two sugar molecules). These break down as follows:

1. **Monosaccharides:** The two most common monosaccharides are glucose and *fructose*:

   Glucose: Most carbs we eat are broken down into glucose, the blood sugar that provides the most important energy source for our bodies. We don't need to obtain glucose from food sources, but foods that naturally contain it include honey, agave, molasses, and fruit (especially dried). It's also found in processed foods such as soda, bottled sauces and salad dressings, energy bars, cereals, cakes, and pies.

Fructose: Found in foods like honey and fruit, fructose is handled differently by your body than other sugars and is metabolized directly by the liver. Unlike glucose, fructose doesn't necessarily cause blood sugar to rise. Instead, if you consume too much, excess fructose turns into fat stored in your body as *triglycerides.*

2. **Disaccharides:** The two most common disaccharides are *sucrose* (glucose plus fructose) and *lactose* (glucose plus *galactose*):

Sucrose: Commonly known as table sugar, sucrose is a 50/50 blend of glucose and fructose. The glucose portion affects your blood sugar, while the fructose part affects your blood fats.

Lactose: A combination of glucose plus galactose, lactose is found in milk products and some processed foods. If you eat more lactose than your body can burn, it ends up stored as fat.

There are more than 60 different names for sugar—easy ones to identify end in "ose" (e.g., dextrose). You may recognize some of these common sugars, which appear often on food labels:

- Agave nectar
- Cane sugar
- Corn syrup
- Fruit juice concentrate
- High-fructose corn syrup
- Honey
- Maple syrup
- Molasses
- Rice syrup

To see a more complete list, visit sugarscience.ucsf.edu /hidden-in-plain-sight.

Starch

When several sugar units bond together, they create starch, a complex carb or polysaccharide. Found primarily in vegetables, grains, and legumes, starch can be difficult to identify because it isn't specifically called out on nutrition labels (see page 60); however, you can determine the amount of starch in a food by subtracting the quantity of sugars and fiber from the total carbs. (If sugar alcohols are listed, subtract them, too.) For example, if a food has 28g of total carbs, 5g of fiber, and 8g of sugar, it contains 28g – 5g – 8g = 15g of starch.

High-starch foods include corn, potatoes, rice, and wheat. With few nutrients and little fiber, refined (i.e., highly processed) starches like white bread and white pasta have a ton of carbs and will increase your blood sugar. On the other hand, foods with a moderate amount of starch include oats, bananas, beans, peas, and lentils. These feature more nutrients and fiber, which are beneficial to your body, though they will increase your blood sugar, too. In other words, if you have diabetes, consume all starches in moderation, favoring those that contain more fiber.

Fiber

Also known as "roughage," fiber is a complex carb your body cannot digest. Found in fruit, vegetables, whole grains, and legumes, fiber helps prevent constipation, lowers your *cholesterol*, and helps you maintain your weight by making you feel full after eating. Best of all, you don't need to count the carbs that come from fiber. In general, fiber falls into two categories:

Insoluble fiber doesn't get digested at all. It helps push food through your GI tract and keeps your colon healthy. Good sources of insoluble fiber include fruit, nuts, seeds, vegetables, and whole grains like brown rice, barley, buckwheat, bulgur, millet, quinoa, and whole-grain varieties of bread, cereal, and pasta.

Soluble fiber dissolves partially during digestion but remains gel-like. It latches onto stuff you don't want around and prevents your body from absorbing anything undesirable or harmful, like cholesterol and cancer-causing toxins. Soluble fiber also slows the rate at which glucose moves into your bloodstream. Good sources of soluble fiber include beans, lentils, peas, fruit, oats, nuts, seeds, and vegetables.

How Much Fiber Should I Eat?

The U.S. Food and Drug Administration's (FDA) recommended Daily Value of fiber is a minimum of 25g for a 2,000-calorie diet. An average person in the United States eats 10 to 13 grams of fiber each day, roughly half the recommended amount. Your body may benefit from more or less fiber, depending on your specific calorie intake, but 25g is a good target.

INSULIN RESISTANCE

Insulin resistance (IR) is a condition in which your body makes insulin but then has trouble using it. Imagine there's a lot of glucose sitting around in your bloodstream waiting for insulin to give it a ride into your cells. Some insulin shows up, but the parts of your body that need glucose don't acknowledge it. Your body therefore signals the beta cells in your pancreas to make even more insulin, and the beta cells fight to keep up. If they succeed, your blood sugar goes down and all is well. If, on the other hand, the beta cells get too tired over time, your pancreas can't keep pace with your body's insulin demands, and prediabetes or type 2 results.

Insulin resistance doesn't have many symptoms, but some people notice dark spots on their skin, especially at the back of the neck. Dark patches may also show up in folds of skin, under the arms, or in the groin area. This condition is known as *acanthosis nigricans*.

What causes insulin resistance isn't totally clear, but researchers suspect a link to excess weight (especially abdominal fat) and physical inactivity. When you exercise regularly, your muscles become more sensitive to insulin. This helps them absorb glucose without having to make that second call to the pancreas for additional insulin. The more muscle your body contains, the better it's able to burn glucose.

So what's a good way to manage your diet and lose weight to counter insulin resistance? Carb counting and exercise. If you have been told you are insulin resistant, use the advice in this book to better manage your blood sugar. Don't put it off until later: Take control of the situation before you get a type 2 diagnosis.

PREDIABETES

Prediabetes results when *blood glucose* is higher than normal, but not elevated enough for a diagnosis of diabetes. Your doctor may request an *oral glucose tolerance test* (OGTT): You drink something containing a large amount of glucose, then your blood sugar is taken at several times over the next few hours to see how quickly the glucose leaves your bloodstream. After the test, your doctor may tell you that you have *impaired fasting glucose* (IFG) or *impaired glucose tolerance* (IGT), but those are just technical terms for prediabetes.

The Centers for Disease Control and Prevention (CDC) estimate that 84 million American adults (one of every three) have prediabetes. The scary part is that 90 percent of them don't know it. Risk factors for prediabetes include:

- Being over the age of 45

- Being overweight

- Coming from certain ethnic backgrounds (African Americans, Alaska Natives, Hispanics/Latinos, American Indians, Pacific Islanders, and some Asian Americans are higher risk)

- Having a parent or sibling with type 2 diabetes

- Having *gestational diabetes* while pregnant and/or giving birth to a baby weighing more than nine pounds

- Having *polycystic ovary syndrome* (PCOS)

- Not being physically active

People with prediabetes may avoid developing type 2 diabetes later in life by committing to lifestyle changes right away. The American Diabetes Association (ADA) reports that people with prediabetes can reduce their risk of developing type 2 by a whopping 58 percent if they:

- Lose 5 to 7 percent of their body weight (that would be 10 to 14 pounds for someone who currently weighs 200 pounds)

- Exercise moderately 30 minutes per day, five days per week

If you have prediabetes, carb counting with the techniques in this book is a great way to control blood sugar and lose weight. A proactive approach will help keep type 2 at bay.

HYPOGLYCEMIA

When the amount of glucose in your bloodstream drops too low, it's called *hypoglycemia*. This condition requires immediate attention, as it can be life-threatening. Hypoglycemia occurs when you take insulin or medications that cause your body to produce more insulin, but you don't pair this with the proper amount of food or activity. As a result, the extra insulin whisks the glucose out of your bloodstream just a little too well.

How to Recognize Hypoglycemia

If someone has a mild to moderate case of hypoglycemia, they may experience any of the following symptoms:

- Anxiety/nervousness
- Being argumentative
- Confusion
- Crying out while sleeping
- Difficulty concentrating
- Dizziness
- Extreme fatigue
- Headache
- Heart palpitations
- Hunger
- Irregular heartbeat
- Irritability
- Pale skin
- Shakiness
- Sweating
- Weakness

If hypoglycemia is not treated, the situation will become dire. A person with severe hypoglycemia may appear to be intoxicated and may also experience:

- Inability to eat or drink
- Inability to complete routine tasks
- A seizure
- Loss of consciousness

How to Treat Hypoglycemia

Treating hypoglycemia involves eating simple carbs (sugar) until your blood glucose returns to a normal range of 70 to 110 mg/dL (milligrams per deciliter). If you suspect your blood sugar is too low, check it with a glucose meter. If the meter confirms that your blood sugar is indeed too low, follow this process:

1. Eat something fast-acting that contains approximately 15g carbs such as:

- 4 glucose tablets
- ½ cup fruit juice (*not* low-calorie or low-carb)
- ½ can soda (*not* low-calorie or low-carb)
- 3 rolls Smarties®
- 1 tablespoon honey or sugar

2. Wait 15 minutes and check your blood sugar again.

3. If your blood sugar is still below 70 mg/dL, repeat this process.

Causes of Hypoglycemia

Hypoglycemia occurs when there is too much insulin in the bloodstream. This can happen when (1) too much insulin is injected, (2) you don't eat as much as usual, or (3) you exercise more than usual. It can also be caused by oral type 2 diabetes medications *sulfonylureas* (glipizide) and *meglitinides* (Prandin®). Other factors that may contribute to hypoglycemia include:

- Drinking too much alcohol without eating food
- Having an illness that prevents you from keeping food down
- Not eating enough carbs
- Skipping or delaying a meal

One way to make sure you are eating the right amount of carbs is to count them. Use the tips in this book to help avoid experiencing hypoglycemia.

MEDICATION

People with type 1 diabetes require insulin therapy. Of those with type 2 diabetes, some manage to keep their blood sugar in range by making lifestyle changes in diet and exercise, while others may need to supplement with diabetes medications or insulin therapy.

Insulin Therapy

People with type 1 diabetes and some with type 2 have pancreases that no longer produce insulin, so they need to provide their body with insulin to stay alive. Insulin is usually injected into fat under the skin using an insulin pump, insulin pen, or syringe. The types of insulin treatment vary according to the following factors:

Onset: How quickly it begins working

Peak: When it's working at maximum potential

Duration: How long its effects last

All insulins come with the risk of hypoglycemia if you use them without the appropriate amount of dietary carbs and exercise. Side effects are rare, but some people are allergic to specific types of insulin and may experience itching, swelling, or redness near the injection site. Here are the categories of available insulin therapies, along with how they break down according to onset, peak, and duration:

Rapid-acting insulin: Begins working in 5 to 15 minutes and only lasts 3 to 4 hours; it reaches its peak in 45 to 75 minutes. Rapid-acting insulin is usually taken just before a meal. Insulin pumps rely exclusively on rapid-acting insulin.

Common names: insulin lispro (Humalog®), insulin aspart (NovoLog®, Fiasp®), insulin glulisine (Apidra®)

Short-acting insulin: Starts working in 30 to 45 minutes, lasts 6 to 8 hours, and reaches its peak in 2 to 4 hours. Short-acting insulin is usually taken about 30 minutes before meals.

Common names: insulin regular (Humulin® R, Novolin® R)

Intermediate-acting insulin: Begins taking effect in 2 hours, lasts 16 to 24 hours, and reaches its peak 4 to 12 hours after injection. Intermediate-acting insulins are used to handle high blood sugar once rapid-acting or short-acting insulin wears off. You can take these either once or twice a day.

Common names: insulin NPH (Humulin® N, Novolin® N)

Long-acting insulin: Starts working in 2 hours and lasts 14 to 24 hours; it has no clear peak. Long-acting insulins lower blood glucose once rapid-acting or short-acting insulin wears off. You can take these once or twice a day.

Common names: insulin glargine (Lantus®, Toujeo®), insulin detemir (Levemir®)

Premixed insulin: Becomes effective in 10 to 30 minutes and lasts 14 to 24 hours. It reaches its peak anywhere from 30 minutes to 12 hours after injection. Premixed insulins combine intermediate-acting and short-acting insulins in one bottle or insulin pen.

Common names: Humulin® 70/30, Novolin® 70/30, NovoLog® Mix 70/30, Humalog® Mix 75/25™

Inhaled insulin: This is a noninjectable type of rapid-acting insulin that peaks in about 20 minutes and completely clears your body in 2 to 3 hours.

Common name: Afrezza®

Type 2 Medications

Blood sugar–lowering type 2 diabetes medications are grouped into classes according to the way they work in your body. Your doctor may prescribe a single pill, multiple pills, or newer combination pills that merge two types of drugs. There is also a newer class of medications, *GLP-1 receptor agonists*, which must be injected.

Biguanides make your body tissues more sensitive to insulin and reduce the amount of glucose produced by your liver. Metformin is usually the first medication in this class prescribed to treat type 2. It may cause intestinal distress when you first start taking it, but these side effects usually wear off over time. For those who can't tolerate metformin, an extended-release version is available that is easier on the digestive system.

Common names: metformin (Glucophage®, Glucophage XR®, Glumetza®, Riomet®, Fortamet®)

Possible side effects: diarrhea, nausea, gas, bloating, lactic acidosis, vitamin B12 deficiency

Risk of hypoglycemia: low

DPP-4 inhibitors block the action of the enzyme *dipeptidyl peptidase-4* (DPP-4) in your body. When you eat, hormones called *incretins* signal your body to release insulin. DPP-4 removes incretins from your body, which is perfectly fine for people who don't have diabetes. However, some people with type 2 don't produce enough incretins and therefore benefit from DPP-4 inhibitor medications, which block the action of DPP-4 and allow the incretins to do their job. These drugs may also be referred to as gliptins.

Common names: sitagliptin (Januvia®), saxagliptin (Onglyza®), linagliptin (Tradjenta®), alogliptin (Nesina®)

Possible side effects: joint pain, respiratory infections, headaches, skin rashes, swelling, urinary tract infections, increased risk for developing pancreatitis, stomach pain

Risk of hypoglycemia: low

GLP-1 receptor agonists mimic the actions of *glucagon-like peptide-1* (GLP-1), one of the incretin hormones that signal your body to release insulin. When you eat, GLP-1 is released from your intestine to make you feel full and slow the rate at which your stomach empties. GLP-1 receptor agonists may help you lose weight, improve your blood pressure and lipids, protect the beta cells in your pancreas, and reduce your chances of having a heart attack. These medications must be injected.

Common names: exenatide (Byetta®, Bydureon®), liraglutide (Victoza®), dulaglutide (Trulicity®), semaglutide (Ozempic®), lixisenitide (Adlyxin®)

Possible side effects: nausea, diarrhea, vomiting, dizziness, headache, increased risk for developing pancreatitis, decreased appetite, indigestion, thyroid tumors

Risk of hypoglycemia: low

Meglitinides, or glinides, are similar to sulfonylureas, but they act much more quickly. Whereas sulfonylureas cause your pancreas to release insulin over a period of several hours, meglitinides stimulate short bursts of insulin to cover meals.

Common names: repaglinide (Prandin®), nateglinide (Starlix®)

Possible side effects: low blood sugar, weight gain, gastrointestinal distress, respiratory infections, back pain

Risk of hypoglycemia: high

SGLT2 inhibitors allow your kidneys to excrete excess glucose through your urine. When you have too much glucose circulating in your bloodstream, your kidneys attempt to remove it from your body. *Sodium-glucose co-transporter 2* (SGLT2) is a protein that tries to preserve the glucose and return it to your bloodstream. In someone with diabetes, this is not desirable. SGLT2 inhibitor drugs, also known as gliflozins, block the effects of SGLT2; this enables the kidneys to remove glucose from the body, resulting in lower blood sugar levels.

Common names: canagliflozin (Invokana®), dapagliflozin (Farxiga®), empagliflozin (Jardiance®), ertugliflozin (Steglatro®)

Possible side effects: yeast infections, urinary tract infections, frequent urination, high potassium, increased cholesterol (LDL), kidney problems, low blood pressure, lower limb amputations, ketoacidosis, bone fractures

Risk of hypoglycemia: low

Sulfonylureas stimulate the beta cells in your pancreas to release insulin and help the body use insulin more effectively. Because these medications have been around for more than 70 years, they are divided into "first generation" and "second generation" versions. First generation sulfonylureas are rarely prescribed now because second generation versions are better at reducing blood sugar and have fewer side effects.

Common names: glipizide (Glucotrol®, Glucotrol XL®), glimepiride (Amaryl®), glyburide (DiaBeta®, Micronase®, Glynase®)

Possible side effects: low blood sugar, weight gain, skin rash, nausea, sensitivity to sunlight, cardiovascular risk

Risk of hypoglycemia: high

Thiazolidinediones increase your body's ability to respond to insulin by reducing insulin resistance. They are referred to as insulin sensitizers or glitazones. Thiazolidinediones also decrease the amount of glucose made by your liver.

Common names: pioglitazone (Actos®), rosiglitazone (Avandia®)

Possible side effects: fluid retention, edema, weight gain, increased body fat, respiratory infections, headache, congestive heart failure, bladder cancer, fractures, increased cholesterol (LDL)

Risk of hypoglycemia: low

Note: Rosiglitazone had been linked to increased risk for heart attack and was removed from the market by the FDA in 2010. After reviewing the results of the RECORD trial in 2013, the FDA concluded that rosiglitazone posed no more of a heart attack risk than other diabetes medications, and it was put back on the market.

Combination medications are now offered as a way to cut back on the number of pills you take each day, which may help you reduce costs. You might see metformin added to an SGLT2 inhibitor or a DPP-4 inhibitor paired with a thiazolidinedione. Keep in mind that these combinations feature the potential benefits as well as the side effects of both drugs. So if you have trouble tolerating metformin, you'll have trouble with any medication that includes it, too.

Common names: metformin and glipizide (Metaglip®), rosiglitazone and glimepiride (Avandaryl®), pioglitazone and metformin (ACTOplus Met®), metformin and glyburide (Glucovance®), rosiglitazone and metformin (Avandamet®), empagliflozin and linagliptin (Glyxambi®), canagliflozin and metformin (Invoka-met®), pioglitazone and glimepiride (Duetact®)

Possible side effects: varied, see lists for specific classes of drugs

Risk of hypoglycemia: varied

Other classes of medications for treatment of type 2 diabetes exist, but they are not commonly prescribed, such as alpha-glucosidase inhibitors, bile acid sequestrants, and dopamine receptor agonists.

Keep in mind that the list of FDA-approved insulins and diabetes medications changes regularly. To see the most up-to-date list, visit www.fda.gov/ForPatients/Illness/Diabetes /ucm408682.htm.

Most important, while insulin therapy and the diabetes medications listed in this chapter can be extremely helpful, you can dial up their effectiveness even further by controlling the amount and type of carbs you eat. The carb-counting tools in this book will help.

CHAPTER TWO

Foods with Carbs

RECOGNIZING CARBS

Now that we understand the importance of carbs to the functioning of our bodies, let's spend some time learning how to recognize carbs in the foods we eat. Most foods contain carbs. So many foods contain them, in fact, that it might be easier to identify the types that *don't*. Foods with no carbs include meat, poultry, eggs, and seafood. Fats like butter and olive oil are carb-free, too.

If I asked you to name a high-carb food, what would you say? I'm guessing you'd pick pasta, potatoes, rice, bread, or some type of dessert. But did you know milk products include carbs, too? Even vegetables like leafy greens and broccoli have them. Here's a more complete list of the types of foods that contain carbs:

- **Dairy products:** cheese, cottage cheese, milk, yogurt
- **Fruits:** all fruits (raw or dried), fruit juices
- **Grains:** barley, bread, cereal, couscous, crackers, oats, pasta, quinoa, rice, rye

- **Nonstarchy vegetables:** artichokes, asparagus, broccoli, Brussels sprouts, cabbage, carrots, cauliflower, eggplant, green beans, leafy greens, mushrooms, tomatoes
- **Starchy vegetables:** beans, corn, lentils, peas, potatoes, sweet potatoes, winter squash
- **Sweet foods:** cakes, candy, chocolate, cookies, doughnuts, pastries, pies, regular soda

Which are the best foods to eat if you are carb counting? In general, you'll want to load up on nonstarchy vegetables. Not only do they have fewer carbs than the other foods on the list, but they also contain critical vitamins and minerals. In addition, you'll want to restrict the amount of sugary foods you eat, as these are extremely high in carbs and have little nutritional bang for the buck.

Here are a few guidelines to follow when deciding which carbs to choose:

Avoid sugar. Eliminate or greatly reduce the number of sweet treats you consume. Make fresh fruit your dessert of choice.

Avoid grains and starchy vegetables at the same meal. Select one of the two unless your portions of each are tiny. Both should fit into one-quarter of your plate.

Choose whole grains that are high in fiber. Avoid foods containing white flour like white bread and pasta, and instead opt for higher-fiber grains such as brown rice, quinoa, and minimally processed oats (e.g., steel-cut). Breads, pastas, and crackers made from 100 percent whole grains may be okay for some people in moderation, while others may not tolerate them at all. Check the ingredient lists of high-grain foods to see if they contain 100 percent whole grains.

Fill up on nonstarchy vegetables. Visit farmers' markets and pick out some locally grown vegetables you've never eaten before. The growers will be thrilled to suggest recipes and may even offer you samples.

Pick starchy vegetables full of protein and/or nutrients. Eat a sweet potato instead of a russet potato for a shot of the *antioxidant* beta-carotene. Choose beans and lentils, which will give you a boost of protein, rather than corn.

Select fresh fruit instead of dried fruit or fruit juice. If you can't live without your morning glass of OJ, squeeze it yourself to avoid the added sugar.

Watch out for flavored yogurt. Even if the yogurt is low-fat or nonfat, the "flavor" comes from sugar. Instead, buy plain Greek yogurt and stir in some fresh or defrosted berries.

PROTEIN AND FAT

Have you reached carb overload yet? In your brain, I mean. Let's put carbs aside for a moment and consider the other two macronutrients: protein and fat.

What Is Protein?

Protein creates, maintains, and repairs the tissues and cells in your body that make up your organs, muscles, skin, bones, hair, and immune system. Your body uses the protein you eat in foods such as beef, pork, chicken, turkey, seafood, eggs, cheese, beans, lentils, and soy to perform specific tasks. Protein is essential, for example, for manufacturing the *hemoglobin* that distributes oxygen throughout your body. It also creates vital chemicals such as *hormones* and *enzymes*. You must eat protein every day, because your body doesn't store it the way it stores glucose.

Much like your small intestine converts carbs into glucose, it also converts protein into *amino acids*. Your body requires 22 amino acids and can generate 13 of them itself. The remaining nine *essential amino acids,* however, you must get from the foods you eat. Animal sources of protein contain all of these essential amino acids, so they're said to be "complete." On the other hand, each plant source of protein is "incomplete," meaning it lacks at least one essential amino acid. Therefore, if you rely on plant-based proteins, make sure you eat a wide variety to guarantee you're getting all the amino acids your body needs.

How much protein should you consume each day? In general, the quality of the protein you eat greatly outweighs the quantity. A 20-year study investigating the impact of low-carb diets on women found that those who ate a diet high in plant sources of protein and fat reduced their risk of type 2 diabetes, while those who ate a diet low in carbs and high in animal sources of protein did not reduce this risk. The ADA says there is no magic bullet for what percentages of your daily calories should come from carbs, fat, and protein. Each person's case is different, and the amount of protein that an individual needs will vary. It does appear to be beneficial, however, to spread out your protein intake throughout the day, rather than eating it all at once.

Healthy Proteins

What are the healthiest proteins? Most dietitians recommend the following:

- Eggs (in moderation) and egg whites
- Fish
- Lean cuts of red meat (occasionally)
- Legumes (beans, lentils, etc.)
- Shellfish (shrimp, scallops, etc.)
- Skinless poultry
- Soy products (tofu, edamame, etc.)

What Is Fat?

Fats have several functions: They supply energy to your body, protect your vital organs, and provide insulation to keep you warm. They also aid in the absorption of fat-soluble vitamins like vitamin A, vitamin D, vitamin E, and vitamin K. Digestive juices in your small intestine convert fats into fatty acids.

You have probably heard of two important groups of fatty acids: *omega-6* and *omega-3*. Each group contains an *essential fatty acid* (EFA) that the body cannot manufacture: *linoleic acid* (LA) in the omega-6 family and *alpha-linolenic acid* (ALA) in the omega-3 family. Two other key omega-3 fatty acids, *eicosapentaenoic acid* (EPA) and *docosahexaenoic acid* (DHA) can be made from ALA, but it's a long process. In general, it's better to get EPA and DHA from food. In fact, studies have shown a connection between higher dietary intake of omega-3s and a decreased risk of cardiovascular disease. Plus, for people with type 2 diabetes and prediabetes, eating more foods with EPA and DHA may combat insulin resistance and lower triglyceride levels.

What foods contain omega-6 and omega-3 fatty acids?

1. **ALA:** This omega-3 fatty acid is found in canola oil, chia seeds, flaxseeds, flaxseed oil, pumpkin seeds, soybeans, soybean oil, tofu, walnuts, and walnut oil.

2. **EPA and DHA:** These omega-3 fatty acids are found in fatty fish such as herrings, mackerel, salmon, sardines, and trout.

3. **LA:** This omega-6 fatty acid is found in nuts, seeds, and vegetable oils such as canola, corn, safflower, and soybean.

Given the preponderance of omega-6 fatty acids in vegetable oils and processed foods, you probably get enough LA already through your diet—you'll do best to concentrate on adding omega-3s.

Fats in your diet fall into several different categories, some of them healthier than others. In general, steer toward unsaturated fats and away from saturated and *trans fats*. The four types of fats are:

1. ***Monounsaturated fats:*** These can lower your cholesterol, thereby reducing your risk of heart disease and stroke. They are also a good source of vitamin E, an antioxidant that

boosts your immune system and keeps your blood vessels healthy. Foods high in monounsaturated fat include avocados, canola oil, olive oil, peanut butter, peanut oil, safflower oil, and sesame oil.

2. *Polyunsaturated fats:* These can also reduce your cholesterol and provide another good source of vitamin E. Oils high in polyunsaturated fat provide your body with the essential fatty acids it cannot produce on its own. Foods containing polyunsaturated fat include plant-based oils such as corn, soybean, and sunflower oil, plus flaxseeds, sunflower seeds, tofu, and walnuts.

3. *Saturated fats:* These can raise your cholesterol and therefore increase your risk of having a heart attack or stroke. Most saturated fats come from animal sources like fatty beef, pork, lamb, poultry skin, lard, cream, butter, cheese, and products made with whole milk. Fried foods and baked goods often contain saturated fat, as well. Plant-based oils like coconut oil and palm oil contain saturated fat, too, but no cholesterol.

4. **Trans fats:** These fats raise your LDL cholesterol (the bad stuff) and lower your HDL cholesterol (the good stuff). Consuming too many trans fats increases your risk of having a heart attack or stroke and also increases your chance of developing type 2 diabetes. Trans fats are primarily found in processed foods like biscuits, frozen pizza, cookies, cake, pie crust, crackers, doughnuts, and stick margarine. The American Heart Association recommends replacing all trans fats in your diet with monounsaturated and polyunsaturated fats.

Here are some dietary recommendations to keep you on track regarding fat:

- Avoid fried foods.
- Eat fatty fish at least twice a week to boost your omega-3s.
- Focus on unsaturated fats.
- Limit your intake of saturated fats.
- Stay away from trans fats.

10 PLACES CARBS HIDE

Since you now have a good handle on recognizing carbs in your diet, let's look at 10 sneaky places where carbs can hide. Carbs also hide in beverages, but we'll examine those in the next section. Before you purchase any of these foods, make sure you check the total carbohydrates on the nutrition label to see if it fits into your eating plan.

1. **Applesauce:** To avoid added sugar, look for unsweetened, unflavored applesauce.

2. **Breakfast cereals:** These foods often include added sugar, while the grains in them bump up the carb count, too. Look for 100 percent whole grains and limited added sugar.

3. **Bottled sauces:** Ketchup, pasta and pizza sauce, and barbecue sauce often contain added sugar.

4. **Canned foods:** Avoid canned fruit stored in syrup, and watch the carb count for soup. One serving (½ cup) of Campbell's® tomato soup, for example, contains 12g of sugar.

5. **Dried fruit:** When water is removed from fresh fruit to dry it out, the sugars in the fruit become concentrated. The result: a lot more sugar in a much smaller package. For instance, ½ cup

of grapes contain about 12g sugar, while ½ cup of raisins has about 49g. Stick with fresh fruit whenever possible.

6. **Flavored yogurt:** As already mentioned, flavored yogurt contains loads of added sugar. One 5.3-ounce container of low-fat strawberry Greek yogurt has 18g carbs, while a similar-sized container of low-fat plain Greek yogurt has less than half that amount—about 8g carbs.

7. **Granola:** This "healthy" food is usually loaded with sugar, maple syrup, or honey. Single servings of some granola contain as much sugar as a slice of cake.

8. **Instant oatmeal:** Most packets and cups of instant oatmeal contain added sugar. One packet of Quaker® Maple and Brown Sugar instant oatmeal has 32g carbs, including 12g sugar.

9. **Protein bars:** Carb counts vary wildly, so look for brands that fit your meal plan.

10. **Salad dressing:** Low-fat and nonfat versions especially tend to contain added sugar.

It's easy to make low-carb versions of most of these foods at home. A slow cooker works well for making homemade ketchup, barbecue sauce, pasta sauce, applesauce, soup, and steel-cut oats. For a tasty vinaigrette, simply shake up oil, vinegar, herbs, and spices in a Mason jar. You can even make your own low-sugar granola and protein bars.

BEVERAGES

Carbs hide in drinks, too—all kinds of drinks. Sweetened beverages can contain more carbs in a single serving than some people with diabetes eat for an entire meal. They don't offer much nutritional value, either. Here are a few you might want to avoid:

- Fruit juice and fruit-flavored drinks
- Lattes and other sweetened coffee drinks
- Regular soda
- Smoothies
- Sports/energy drinks
- Sweetened iced tea

If you decide to indulge in sugary drinks, make sure you know their carb counts and factor them into your daily meal plan. For example, 12 ounces of regular soda or sweet tea is in the 35 to 40g carb range. A 12-ounce Starbucks® Caffè Vanilla Light Frappuccino® (nonfat milk, no whipped cream) contains 29g sugar (30g total carbs), and a small Jamba Juice® Peanut Butter Moo'd® Smoothie clocks in at a whopping 72g sugar (83g total carbs). Even a supposedly "healthy" 8-ounce energy drink or glass of orange juice contains about 27g carbs.

Healthy beverage choices include water, unsweetened tea, and black coffee. To jazz up plain water, try infusing it with citrus fruits (oranges, limes, or lemons), cucumber, strawberries, or mint—cucumber and mint make an especially refreshing combination. If you're feeling really creative, try hibiscus flowers and goji berries. Interesting flavors of tea can also make delicious hot or cold drinks, no sugar required. Try brewing your own loose-leaf tea for more variety. Loose tea and tea bags come in regular and decaffeinated versions. Green tea, full of antioxidants, is one of the healthiest beverages you can drink. When I was first diagnosed with diabetes, I switched from coffee in the morning to green tea. (I can drink tea without a sweetener, but not coffee.)

SUGAR SUBSTITUTES

If you prefer, you can use artificial sweeteners (a.k.a. sugar substitutes). There are several sugar substitutes available that contain few or no carbs, so they have a minimal effect on blood sugar. I avoid them because they make me crave sweet foods, but your mileage may vary. However, at least one new study shows a possible link between using artificial sweeteners and weight gain, believe it or not.

To date, the FDA has approved six artificial sweeteners:

1. **Acesulfame potassium (Ace-K):** Sweet One®, Sunett®

2. **Advantame**

3. **Aspartame:** NutraSweet®, Equal®, Sugar Twin®

4. **Neotame:** Newtame®

5. **Saccharin:** Sweet'N Low®, Sweet Twin®, Necta Sweet®

6. **Sucralose:** Splenda®

The FDA has also given the generally recognized as safe (GRAS) designation to two other plant-based sugar substitutes:

1. **Luo Han Guo fruit extracts (monk fruit):** Nectresse®, Monk Fruit in the Raw®, PureLo®

2. **Steviol glycosides (stevia):** Truvia®, Pure Via™, Enliten®

Sugar Alcohols

Another category of sweeteners is known as *sugar alcohol*. Unlike the previously listed substitutes, sugar alcohols contain carbs. However, these carbs digest slowly and have less of an impact on blood glucose than other sugars do. To recognize sugar alcohols, look for an "ol" at the end; *sorbitol, xylitol, maltitol, lactitol, mannitol*, and *erythritol* are all sugar alcohols. However, some don't end in "ol," such as *isomalt* and *hydrogenated starch hydrolysates* (HSH). Sugar alcohols are found in sugar-free baked goods, frozen desserts, candies, cough syrups, throat lozenges, chewing gum, and chocolate-flavored coatings. One important thing to remember about sugar alcohols: They can have a laxative effect, so consume these in moderation.

ALCOHOL

Alcohol may be fine in small amounts for some people with diabetes, but not for everyone. Drinking alcohol can make your blood sugar drop too low, especially if you take insulin or type 2 medications that can cause hypoglycemia. Your liver works so hard to get the alcohol out of your system that it forgets to manage your blood sugar. Ask your health care team if drinking alcohol is safe for your particular case.

If you get the go-ahead to drink, keep the following tips in mind:

- **Check your blood sugar before having a drink:** Never consume alcohol when your blood sugar is already low.

- **Don't drink on an empty stomach:** Always have something to eat when you drink alcohol.

- **Check your blood sugar before bed:** If you drink alcohol in the evening, check your blood sugar before you go to sleep. If it's trending low, you may need to eat a snack.

- **Remember your best drink options:** Dry wine and hard liquor with low-sugar mixers are your best options, carb-wise.

- **Keep serving sizes in mind:** Remember that one serving of wine is 5 fluid ounces and one serving of liquor is 1½ fluid ounces.

- **Count the carbs in sweet wine or beer:** One serving is 12 fluid ounces of beer and 5 fluid ounces of wine.

- **Avoid sweet mixers:** Stay away from sugary drinks like rum and regular Coke®, margaritas, and piña coladas.

GLUTEN-FREE

Gluten is a type of protein found in wheat and other grains. When someone with *celiac disease* eats gluten, their immune system responds by attacking their small intestine. Over time, the intestine becomes damaged to the point that it can no longer facilitate the absorption of nutrients into the body, a very serious condition. There is another group of people who don't test positive for celiac disease but are equally sensitive to the effects of wheat. These folks have *non-celiac wheat sensitivity* and experience symptoms similar to those of people with celiac disease.

Currently, the only treatment for both groups is to adopt a gluten-free diet that eliminates wheat, rye, barley, triticale, and some oats. Beyond these conditions, some people feel better when they don't eat wheat because they have less bloating and gas. This is particularly true for people who have *irritable bowel syndrome* (IBS). Others are simply allergic to wheat.

If you have diabetes and wonder if you should adopt a gluten-free diet, consider the following:

- **Celiac disease and type 1 diabetes are both autoimmune diseases:** If you already have one autoimmune disease, research has shown that you are likely to develop another one every 10 years. If you have type 1 diabetes, you may want to get tested for celiac disease and wheat sensitivity.

- **Gluten-free does not mean carb-free or even low-carb:** Some gluten-free foods have fewer nutrients but more carbs, saturated fat, and sodium than their gluten-filled counterparts. Always read labels.

- **No proven link exists between celiac disease and type 2 diabetes:** People with type 2 diabetes have about the same chance of developing celiac disease as people without diabetes. So far, no connection has been established between type 2 and gluten sensitivity.

RECOMMENDED CARB COUNTERS

I intentionally do not include an exhaustive list of carb counts and other nutritional data for specific foods in this book, since many other excellent resources provide this type of information. Whether you prefer carb counters in the form of apps, online databases, or books, here are a few popular options:

CalorieKing is an app, a website (calorieking.com), and a book (*The CalorieKing Calorie, Fat, and Carbohydrate Counter,* by Allan Borushek). The app is currently available only on iPhone, but an Android version is in development. I have actually seen suggestions in the diabetes online community (DOC) for people to switch from Android to iPhone just to be able to use the CalorieKing app! CalorieKing began as a book, first published in Australia in 1973 and is still updated every year. The free iPhone app allows you to search for foods by category, food item, or brand, and includes menu items at more than 250 chain restaurants. You can also adjust the serving size on the fly. For example, if a serving size is 45g and you plan to eat 2 ounces, it will do the conversion for you, no math required. CalorieKing is purely a food database.

ControlMyWeight is a relatively new app from the CalorieKing folks that offers more MyFitnessPal-like features. You enter your height, weight, age, and activity level, and it picks a goal for you ("maintain weight," in my case). Then it tells you how many calories you need each day to reach that goal and asks you to set a target for how many minutes you'll exercise each day. When you visit your food diary, you see how many calories you've consumed toward your allotment, and how many more minutes you need to exercise (only if you've logged them, of course). Entering a recipe seems to be easier than on MyFitnessPal (page 33), and I have more confidence in the nutrition information.

Lose It! is both an app and a website (loseit.com) and is similar in functionality to MyFitnessPal and ControlMyWeight. You enter your birthday, height, weight, sex, and goal weight, and it will give you a daily calorie budget. You can then enter what you eat and your type of exercise, and it will track for you. One thing I really like is that Lose It! shows that you actually burn calories when you lift weights (MyFitnessPal doesn't). One unique feature is that you can take a photo with your phone of a barcode, and Lose It! will add that food to your diary, complete with nutritional information. Theoretically, you can also take a photo of a food you're about to eat, and it will identify and log it for you. My test with a spaghetti squash, however, was less than successful (Lose It! suggested I had a lemon, mango, or cheesecake). Many people like Lose It! because the app syncs with their fitness trackers and other devices.

MyFitnessPal is an app and a website (myfitnesspal.com); the app is available in both iPhone and Android versions. I use MyFitness-Pal to calculate nutritional information for my own recipes, to look up menu items when I'm going to a particular restaurant, and to log my exercise (MyFitnessPal syncs with fitness trackers). It also has a feature where you can type in the URL of an online recipe and it will give you the carb count and other nutrient information. MyFitnessPal allows you to set your target calories for each day and then breaks down the percentage of calories from carbs, fat, and protein. On any given day, you can see a pie chart that lets you know how you're doing in real time. If you have trouble drinking enough water, you can track that, too. When I have a particularly good blood sugar day, I print out my diary log, and I have a meal plan for future use. One thing to beware of when using MyFitnessPal is that users can enter their own data about certain foods, so you have to be careful when searching entries to pick ones that have been verified.

The Complete Book of Food Counts: The Book That Counts It All, by Corinne T. Netzer, is the gold standard when it comes to carb-counting reference books. When I was diagnosed with type 2 in 1999, there were no smartphones and not many nutrition-based websites, so I used Netzer's book extensively to track my carbs. This book is essentially one giant alphabetical list of foods. You don't have to worry about what category something might be in (is orange juice a *fruit* or a *beverage*?), just look up "orange juice" under "O"; you'll also find the breakdown of calories, protein, carbs, fat, cholesterol, sodium, and fiber for foods produced by various brands. Interested in carb counts for restaurant foods? Look up the restaurant's name, not the food. If you prefer to track things with pencil and paper, this is the resource for you. The bad news? The book hasn't been updated since 2011, and you'll have to bone up on your math skills.

USDA Food Composition Database (ndb.nal.usda.gov/ndb) serves as the engine for most of the carb-counting websites and apps. Accessing the database directly from the website isn't as much fun or as user-friendly as an app, but you get the information you need. You can search the entire database or limit your search to "Branded Food Products" or "Standard Reference." The standard report shows calories, carbs, protein, fat, fiber, vitamins, minerals, and fatty acids. The full report provides a more complete list of nutrients, including a category for amino acids. You can even download the reports generated on various foods in CSV or PDF format. (This is the place for nutrient geeks.) Just note: When you do a search, scroll inside the sub-window that pops up to see all the information. At first, only a few lines will be visible, but don't assume that's all there is.

PART II

Handy Tools for Counting Carbs

Now that you understand how the carbs you consume turn into the glucose that fuels your body, as well as how to recognize carbs in food, we can finally turn to the main issue: determining how many carbs to eat each day. We'll start with an estimate, and then explain how to fine-tune that with personal details—and a bit of experimentation—to achieve the best possible blood sugar management for your individual case.

Chapter 3 will provide simple strategies for calculating your daily carb allowance, teach you how to handle special occasions when you may eat more or fewer carbs than usual, and offer ways to experiment with your carb intake to make sure you are getting the optimal blood sugar results for your particular circumstances.

Chapter 4 will explain why carbs are measured in grams and how to make sure you are eating appropriate portions of food. You'll also learn tips for accurately estimating portion sizes for those situations when you can't measure, and how to time your carb consumption throughout the day.

Chapter 5 will give some alternatives to carb counting, including avoiding "white" foods, using the *plate method*, and "eating the rainbow."

Chapter 6 will teach you how to read a nutrition label, as well as the significance of *glycemic index* (GI) and *glycemic load* (GL). You'll also discover a few ways to improve your carb-counting accuracy.

Chapter 7 will cover meal planning. You'll learn why you should plan meals in advance, and I'll provide examples of weekly and daily meal plans, including ways to make the process less cumbersome.

Finally, chapter 8 discusses the importance of being honest with yourself when carb counting, and offers several methods for tracking your carb intake.

CHAPTER THREE

Setting Your Target

HOW MANY CARBS?

The big question is how many carbs should you eat each day? The answer, unfortunately, is that it varies—wildly. Your age, sex, body size, weight goals, level of physical activity, and length of time you've been living with diabetes all play into the equation. The ADA's nutrition therapy recommendations state that "evidence is inconclusive for an ideal amount of carbohydrate intake for people with diabetes." Therefore, your best bet for coming up with an optimal eating plan for your particular situation is to work with a *certified diabetes educator* (CDE) or *registered dietitian* (RD).

Unfortunately, for many people, consulting a CDE or RD just isn't an option. Folks in rural areas may not have one nearby, and for others, the cost may be prohibitive. So if you'd like to tackle this on your own, here are some general guidelines.

Find Your Recommended Calorie Intake

Before you try to figure out the correct number of carbs to eat each day, you'll need to know how many calories you should be consuming. You can estimate this from a chart or use an interactive online tool.

Technique #1

To estimate your daily calorie budget, refer to the following charts adapted from the health.gov website. The first chart is for women, the second for men. Find your age in the far-left column, then scan over to the activity level that best represents you. "Sedentary" means you don't get any exercise beyond what it takes to live independently. "Moderately Active" means you walk 1.5 to 3 miles per day at a rate of 3 to 4 miles per hour (or get a similar amount of another type of exercise). "Active" means you walk more than 3 miles per day at a rate of 3 to 4 miles per hour (or get a similar amount of another type of exercise.)

DAILY CALORIE BUDGET FOR WOMEN

AGE	SEDENTARY	MODERATELY ACTIVE	ACTIVE
18	1,800	2,000	2,400
19–25	2,000	2,200	2,400
26–30	1,800	2,000	2,400
31–50	1,800	2,000	2,200
51–60	1,600	1,800	2,200
61+	1,600	1,800	2,000

DAILY CALORIE BUDGET FOR MEN

AGE	SEDENTARY	MODERATELY ACTIVE	ACTIVE
18	2,400	2,800	3,200
19–20	2,600	2,800	3,000
21–25	2,400	2,800	3,000
26–35	2,400	2,600	3,000
36–40	2,400	2,600	2,800
41–45	2,200	2,600	2,800
46–55	2,200	2,400	2,800
56–60	2,200	2,400	2,600
61–65	2,000	2,400	2,600
66–75	2,000	2,200	2,600
76+	2,000	2,200	2,400

According to the first chart, a 55-year-old woman who walks a couple of miles a day at a decent pace would need 1,800 calories daily to maintain her current weight. If she wanted to lose weight at a healthy rate (approximately one pound per week), she should reduce her daily calorie intake by 500 for a total of 1,300 calories. Similarly, if she wanted to gain a pound a week, she should increase her calories to 2,300 per day.

Technique #2

While technique #1 considers sex, age, and activity level, it doesn't take into account your current weight. Clearly, an active 40-year-old man weighing 240 pounds will require more calories to maintain his weight than one weighing 160 pounds. A more accurate way to calculate how many calories you need each day is to use an app or an online tool such as NIDDK's Body Weight Planner, currently found at niddk.nih.gov/health-information/weight-management/body-weight-planner. Using this particular tool, you enter your weight, sex, age, height, activity level, goal weight (and when you want to reach it), and by what percentage you're willing to increase your activity level. It will then tell you how many calories you need to maintain your current weight, how many to reach your goal, and how many to maintain your goal weight. Note that your goal weight and current weight can be the same.

Now Think about Carbs

Now that you know how many calories you should be eating every day, it's time to figure out how many grams of carbs to eat. Unfortunately, this is more confusing than it should be. The Dietary Reference Intakes (DRI), set by the National Academy of Sciences and referenced by many dietitians, recommends a minimum daily carb intake of 45 percent of total calories and a maximum of 65 percent for adults. They say that, no matter what, you should consume at least 130g of carbs per day to keep your brain functioning at its peak. However, newer studies, though small and short-term, are beginning to show that eating fewer carbs may lead to improved blood sugar control and may be fine for brain performance, too. Stay tuned.

People with diabetes often get 45 percent or less of their calories from carbs. The ADA says there's no ideal number regarding daily carb intake for people with diabetes, but their meal plans target 45 percent. While the Joslin Diabetes Center's guideline is 40 percent, they agree with the ADA that you should tailor your individual carb intake to your specific situation. Moderately low-carb eating plans allot 20 to 35 percent of daily calories from carbs, low-carb plans come in at 10 to 20 percent, and extremely low-carb plans like the ketogenic diet suggest 5 to 10 percent. I'd suggest starting with 40 to 45 percent, assessing whether your blood sugars are consistently in range, and then making adjustments as necessary. Remember, everyone is different.

Reference the following chart to see how many grams of carbs you should aim for at various daily calorie levels. Find your calories

CALORIES/DAY	EXTREMELY LOW-CARB 10%	LOW-CARB 20%
1,100	28	55
1,200	30	60
1,300	33	65
1,400	35	70
1,500	38	75
1,600	40	80
1,700	43	85
1,800	45	90
1,900	48	95
2,000	50	100
2,100	53	105
2,200	55	110
2,300	58	115
2,400	60	120
2,500	63	125
2,600	65	130
2,700	68	135
2,800	70	140
2,900	73	145
3,000	75	150

MODERATELY LOW-CARB			JOSLIN	ADA
25%	30%	35%	40%	45%
69	83	96	110	124
75	90	105	120	135
81	98	114	130	146
88	105	123	140	158
94	113	131	150	169
100	120	140	160	180
106	128	149	170	191
113	135	158	180	203
119	143	166	190	214
125	150	175	200	225
131	158	184	210	236
138	165	192	220	248
144	173	201	230	259
150	180	210	240	270
156	188	219	250	281
163	195	228	260	293
169	203	236	270	304
175	210	245	280	315
181	218	254	290	326
188	225	263	300	338

* The DRI does not currently recommend a daily carb intake of less than 130g for any adult.

per day in the left column, then scan over to the percentage of calories you want to get from carbs.

If your exact calorie allocation isn't in the table, you can do the calculation yourself. You'll need to know that 1 gram of carbs contains 4 calories. First, to get the daily total calories from carbs, multiply the calories per day by the percentage you want to come from carbs (e.g., 0.4 for 40 percent). Then divide that number by 4 to get the number of grams.

For example, the Lose It! app says I need 1,659 calories per day. Let's assume I want 40 percent of them to come from carbs:

Daily total calories from carbs:
1659 x 0.4 = 663.6

Daily total carbs (in grams):
663.6 ÷ 4 = 165.9 (round to 166)

FIND YOUR SWEET SPOT

You're now armed with a target number of calories and grams of carbs to eat every day. For most people, it's best to spread out your carbs throughout the day to keep your blood glucose as steady as possible. If you have three meals and two snacks, divide your daily grams of carbs by four to get your carb allowance per meal (note that two snacks equal one meal). Divide that number again in half to get your carb allowance per snack. So using the previous example, I'd be at about 42g per meal (166 ÷ 4) and 21g per snack (42 ÷ 2). How can you tell if these estimates are ideal for you? Just experiment. Here's a general process to follow:

1. Eat a meal containing your target number of carbs.

2. Check your blood glucose (BG) two hours later. (I find it helpful to set a timer on my phone as soon as I start eating.)

3. If your BG is within range, the amount and type of carbs you ate is probably okay for you (at this point in your diabetes journey). If your BG is high, try eating the same amount of carbs, but include more fiber at your next meal. If it's still coming in high, cut back on the amount of carbs. Alternatively, if your BG reads low, you may need to eat more carbs next time or make an adjustment in your medication.

You may also want to check your BG just before you eat. If it was high before your meal and you're at about the same place two hours later, you'll know the meal itself had little effect.

SPECIAL OCCASIONS

Certain life circumstances derail even the best-laid carb-counting plans. Here are a few situations that may impact your blood sugar control:

Age and stage of life: It's not surprising that both of these may impact blood sugar control. Young people have crazy hormones and may need frequent insulin adjustments. Birth control pills (especially ones high in estrogen) may affect insulin response, as well. Menstrual cycles in general can affect blood sugar control, too. Women who are pregnant or breastfeeding may need more carbs than usual, while older folks may need fewer calories, but more nutrient-dense carbs.

Illness and surgery: Both of these factors produce stress hormones that can make your blood sugar increase. Over-the-counter cold and sinus medicines may contain sugar and/or alcohol: The sugar will make blood sugar rise, while the alcohol may cause it to fall. If you have the stomach flu and can't keep anything down, you may need to drink diluted fruit juice, regular soda, or gelatin to keep your blood sugar from dropping too low. Check your BG more often when you're sick. If you have surgery planned, be sure you discuss potential blood sugar impacts beforehand with your doctor.

Parties, holidays, and weddings: These occasions are usually landmines for blood-sugar control. With abundant high-carb appetizers and side dishes, breads, cakes, pies, and free-flowing alcohol, it's tough to stay on track. Your best bet? Look for raw vegetables on the appetizer table, skip the bread, and load up on protein. You can taste everything, just don't eat a full serving of any high-carb food. If you can't resist dessert, pick fruit or scrape the icing off a small piece of cake. (Eat the cake, not the icing.) Another winning strategy is to eat a small meal at home before you go—that way you won't be hungry or feel as tempted.

Stressful situations and high emotions: Both of these can increase blood glucose, so keep a close eye on your blood sugar levels if you are facing tough professional challenges or emotional life events; these might include planning a wedding or a move, dreading an upcoming medical test, facing a huge deadline at work or school, going through a divorce, interviewing for a new job, or worrying about a loved one's health.

Vacations and business travel: Exploring new places can offer opportunities to try different foods, and you may not know how these will affect your blood sugar. Many conferences that include meals don't plan them with diabetic eaters in mind. Your normal eating schedule may be disrupted, too; for example, dinner may be closer to bedtime than you'd like. You may also drink more alcohol when you travel. To monitor possible effects, check your BG more often and make any adjustments you can to your eating habits when you're on the road. Take snacks along with you so you won't be tempted by high-carb foods at the airport. If you have no control over the menu at an event, ask if you can special order a "diabetic-friendly" or "low-carb" meal ahead of time.

CHAPTER FOUR

Measuring Carbs

WHY WE WEIGH CARBS

When I was diagnosed with type 2 diabetes, carb counting wasn't really a thing. Instead, my CDE told me about the exchange system. Foods were broken into the categories of meat, starch, fruit, milk, vegetable, and fat. I followed a plan where I could eat a certain number of each food category each day. I carried around a little notebook that included the correct number of checkboxes beside each exchange type. If I ate a slice of whole-wheat toast with 1 teaspoon butter, a boiled egg, and ¾ cup blueberries for breakfast, I checked off one starch box, one fat box, one meat box, and one fruit box. I had to know that a slice of bread was one "starch," a teaspoon of butter was one "fat," an egg was one "meat," and ¾ cup blueberries was one "fruit." There was a lot to memorize.

The exchange method worked for me—I lost about 35 pounds in six months, and my blood sugars were always in range. In fact, when the "carb counting" craze came along, I resisted the change.

But I finally realized how much easier and more accurate the new system was. Knowing exact carb counts led to even better blood sugar control—especially important as my diabetes progressed.

Carbs are always measured in grams (g), the metric system's unit of weight. Consider a small banana, a.k.a. one fruit exchange. You might define the word *small* differently from your partner (especially if you like bananas more than he or she does). Your "small" might be a 4-ounce banana, while your partner's might be a 3-ounce banana. If each of you ate your bananas, you would consume about 27g carbs while your partner would consume only 19g. More precise data simply leads to better control.

PROPER PORTIONS

If you've eaten out lately (and who hasn't?), you may have noticed that most restaurants serve gargantuan amounts of food. I've gotten to the point where I either just order an appetizer or my husband and I split an entrée. While oversized portions of food may make us feel we're getting a good deal, eating too much is something we need to avoid.

The first step in combatting overload is to identify appropriate portion sizes for the foods we eat and to understand the difference between the terms *serving size* and *portion size*. A serving size is the quantity of a particular food for which the nutrition information has been calculated. If you look at the label for black beans, for example, you'll see a serving size is defined as ½ cup. Meanwhile, a portion size is the amount of the food you actually eat. Therefore, if you eat 1 cup of black beans, your portion will be 2 servings. If 1 serving is listed as 21g carbs, you will have eaten twice that amount (42g).

Identifying serving size is fairly easy if you're eating foods with labels, but what if your diet consists of fresh vegetables, fruit, and meat, as most dietitians recommend? How do you know what appropriate serving sizes are and how many carbs a serving contains? You'll need to look them up. You can use the USDA database or any of the other resources listed in chapter 2.

Serving Sizes for Common Foods

Ideal portion sizes for various foods differ from person to person. They also may vary depending on what other foods you eat at the same time. If you've recently been diagnosed with prediabetes or diabetes, chances are your portion sizes of certain foods (especially high-carb ones) are larger than they should be. Below are a few guidelines on serving sizes for common foods. Note that they may not be the same as the serving sizes defined on nutrition labels.

- **Beans:** ⅓ cup*
- **Berries:** ¾ cup to 1 cup*
- **Bread:** 1 slice (1 ounce)*
- **Cheese:** 1 ounce
- **Cooked oats:** ½ cup*
- **Cooked pasta:** ½ cup*
- **Cooked rice:** ⅓ cup*
- **Fats (e.g., olive oil):** 1 teaspoon
- **Fish, seafood, poultry, meat (cooked):** 3 ounces
- **Milk:** 1 cup
- **Nonstarchy vegetables (raw):** 3 cups*
- **Nonstarchy vegetables (cooked):** 1½ cups*
- **Starchy vegetables:** ½ cup*
- **Yogurt (plain):** ¾ cup

* This serving size contains approximately 15g carbs.

Measure Everything

Invest in a reliable digital kitchen scale, measuring cups, and measuring spoons, and use them often. You may think you know what 3 ounces of fish looks like, but do you really? Test yourself: Portion out what you think ½ cup oatmeal or an ounce of cheese looks like, and then measure it. How close were you? Weigh and measure everything until your "eyeball" measurements are extremely accurate. Check yourself every month or so to avoid "portion creep"—in other words, allowing your portions to grow larger.

One way to make sure your portion sizes align with your meal plan is to premeasure. If you purchase nuts in bulk, ration out appropriate serving sizes into small snack bags. If you buy a big block of cheese, slice it up into 1-ounce portions.

ESTIMATING PORTIONS

Now that you have a handle on how much of certain foods you should be eating, what happens when you're in a situation when you don't have a scale handy or you can't be bothered to measure?

First, get familiar with what an appropriate serving size looks like in your own dinnerware. Measure out ¾ cup of yogurt into one of your own bowls and notice how full (or not) it is. From then on, you'll know how much to put in your bowl, and you won't need to measure. (I recommend you use the smallest bowl that will fit your food; otherwise, you'll feel deprived seeing a dish that seems somewhat empty.) Do this for all of the foods you eat regularly. You can also buy portion-control dinnerware offered by companies like Livliga® and Precise Portions®. The designs on the plates and bowls cleverly disguise hints about appropriate portion sizes.

Next, it's helpful to compare portion sizes to objects you know. Granted, larger people have larger body parts, but in general, use these measurements:

- **One fist is the size of about 1 cup.** Use this for cooked, non-starchy vegetables and milk.
- **One handful is the size of about ½ cup.** This is a good way to estimate serving sizes of pasta, starchy vegetables, and oatmeal. A little less than a handful is about a serving size for beans or rice. A little more than a handful is a serving of berries or yogurt. (Of course, I don't recommend you actually hold the foods.)
- **Two fists are the size of about 2 cups.** This works well for raw vegetables and salads.

- **Your index finger is the size of about 1 ounce.** This is a good estimate for cheese and nuts.
- **Your palm (or a deck of cards) is the size of about 3 ounces of protein.** Use this for chicken, fish, seafood, and meat.
- **Your thumb is the size of about 1 tablespoon.** One-third of your thumb is the size of one serving of fat.

HOW OFTEN?

In general, most people with diabetes have better blood sugar control when they spread their carbs throughout the day. So how do you figure out the right amount carbs to eat at one time? As a starting point, take the number of daily carbs you calculated in chapter 3. For the sake of illustration, let's assume that number is 130g. The following calculations will help you determine how many carbs to include at each meal:

If you eat three meals per day and no snacks
just divide by 3:
carbs per meal: 130 ÷ 3 = 43.3 (round to 43)

If you eat three meals per day plus one snack
first subtract 15g (carbs per snack),
then divide the rest by 3:
carbs per meal: 130 − 15 = 115; 115 ÷ 3 = 38.3 (round to 38)

If you eat three meals per day plus two snacks
divide by 4 (because 2 snacks = 1 meal) to get the amount per meal,
then divide that number in half to get the amount per snack:
carbs per meal: 130 ÷ 4 = 32.5 (round to 33)
carbs per snack: 32.5 ÷ 2 = 16.25 (round to 16)

If you eat six small meals per day
just divide by 6:
carbs per small meal: 130 ÷ 6 = 21.7 (round to 22)

You get the idea. There may be circumstances when you want to vary the number of carbs you eat at different meals. For example, some people find that eating the majority of their carbs early in the day works best. Others experience something called the *dawn phenomenon,* or dawn effect, which can occur in some people with diabetes in the early morning as their body prepares to wake up. Hormones such as cortisol and growth hormone are released, which then trigger the liver to pump out glucose, causing a temporary rise in blood sugar. If this happens to you, you may find that opting for a lower-carb breakfast or dinner works better for you. Personally, if I exercise in the morning, I tend to eat more of my carb allowance at breakfast and lunch. On the other hand, if I exercise in the afternoon, I'll likely have more of my carbs at lunch and dinner.

One important note on the timing of carbs: You'll probably manage your blood sugar more successfully if you don't skip meals. This is because not eating frequently enough can cause hypoglycemia or blood sugar spikes when you finally do eat. However, most people react positively once they get on a regular schedule, eating their meals and snacks at roughly the same time each day. Experiment to see what works best for you.

CHAPTER FIVE

Alternatives to Counting

I love numbers and data. I also enjoy keeping records, but I realize not everyone shares these particular passions. If the thought of having to count, track, add, subtract, multiply, and divide fills you with dread, check out these other methods for keeping your carbs in check, no math required.

AVOID WHITE FOODS

One way to reduce the carbs in your life is to simply avoid eating most foods that are white. For some reason, white foods tend to contain a lot of carbs but lack fiber and nutrients. (Of course, there are notable exceptions, such as cauliflower.) What foods fall into the "white" category?

- **Anything made with sugar (and often white flour, too):** Candy, cookies, cake, pie, pastries, and muffins
- **Anything made with white flour:** Bread, crackers, cereal, pasta, bagels, pretzels, and pizza dough

- **White potatoes:** Russet, gold, new, Red Bliss, and fingerling
- **White rice:** par-boiled, long-grain, short-grain, basmati, jasmine, Arborio, and sushi rice

White flour, sugar, and rice are all refined foods—this means that most of their nutritional benefits are stripped out during processing. In contrast, products made with 100 percent whole grains add fiber and nutrients to your diet, while making you feel full much more quickly. It's a good idea to cut back on flour-based foods in general, but be sure to select versions made with 100 percent whole grains when you do choose to eat them. As far as sugar is concerned, just stay away. The average American consumes more than 19 teaspoons of sugar each day (an astonishing 66 *pounds* a year)—that's more than double the recommended amount. Let the sweetness in your life come from fresh fruit instead.

Sweet potatoes provide delicious, nutrient-dense replacements for white potatoes. As for white rice substitutes, brown rice, quinoa, whole-wheat couscous, bulgur, farro, and millet are all good choices, although you'll still need to watch your serving size, as all of these grains still contain carbs. You can even make "rice" out of cauliflower and eat all you like. Here's a quick and easy recipe for whipping up cauliflower rice:

1. Buzz up a head of cauliflower in a food processor and microwave for 5 minutes at 100 percent.

2. Dump the cauliflower onto a clean dish towel, let it cool for 10 minutes or so, and then wring out as much liquid as possible.

3. Heat olive oil in a skillet and sauté chopped onion, garlic, and ginger.

4. Add the riced cauliflower, heat for about 5 minutes, and season with white pepper.

BALANCE YOUR PLATE

Another way to cut back on carbs without doing any math or tracking is to follow the plate method. I've found controlling portions so much easier if you start with a salad plate (8½ inches in diameter) instead of a larger dinner plate (10 or more inches). Here's the idea:

1. Divide your plate in half, and then divide one side in half again. (Okay, I know I used the word *divide*, but no numbers were involved.) You now have one large section and two smaller sections.

2. Fill the large section with nonstarchy vegetables.

3. Add lean protein to one of the small sections.

4. Place fiber-rich grains and/or nutrient-dense starchy vegetables in the remaining small section.

5. Add some healthy fat like avocado, nuts, seeds, or olive oil.

6. Add dairy and/or fruit on the side, if compatible with your meal plan.

7. Drink water, unsweetened tea, or black coffee.

   Here's what a meal might look like using the plate method:

- **Large section:** spinach salad with roasted red peppers, artichokes, and citrus vinaigrette
- **Smaller section #1:** grilled chicken marinated in olive oil, lemon juice, and Italian herbs
- **Smaller section #2:** wild rice and lentil pilaf
- **On the side:** plain Greek yogurt with fresh berries, slivered almonds, and pumpkin seeds
- **To drink:** unsweetened tea

THE PLATE METHOD

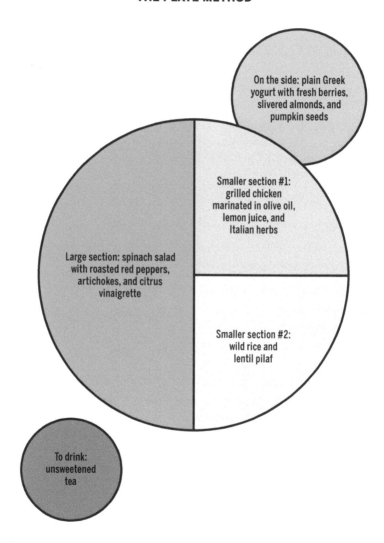

On the side: plain Greek yogurt with fresh berries, slivered almonds, and pumpkin seeds

Smaller section #1: grilled chicken marinated in olive oil, lemon juice, and Italian herbs

Large section: spinach salad with roasted red peppers, artichokes, and citrus vinaigrette

Smaller section #2: wild rice and lentil pilaf

To drink: unsweetened tea

EAT YOUR COLORS

One more way to limit carbs without counting is to focus on eating a "rainbow" of naturally colorful fruits and vegetables. These foods are rich in fiber and important nutrients, yet often low in carbs. You'll find them in a range of vibrant colors, including:

Green: Foods that are green, especially dark green, are often called superfoods due to their knockout nutritional value. Vegetables like Brussels sprouts, spinach, kale, broccoli, mustard greens, and bok choy contain a slew of nutrients like potassium, vitamin C, vitamin E, and folate. Try to eat something green at every meal—even breakfast, if you can. Just doing this one simple thing will greatly improve the quality of your diet.

Orange and yellow: Foods like sweet potatoes, carrots, mangoes, and cantaloupe contain *beta-carotene,* which converts to vitamin A in your body. Vitamin A is important for your vision and to keep your immune system strong. Orange and yellow foods also contain vitamin C, folic acid, and potassium.

Purple and blue: Foods like blueberries and eggplant contain flavonoids, which keep your blood flowing and brain functioning properly.

Red: Foods that are red, like tomatoes, tomato sauce, and watermelon, contain *lycopene*, which may help prevent heart disease and some cancers.

White: Unlike white foods that contain refined sugar and white flour, nonstarchy white vegetables and legumes, like cauliflower, onions, mushrooms, parsnips, fennel, turnips, white beans, and chickpeas, are fine additions to your diet. Though some of these are higher in carbs than others, all contribute important nutrients.

Loading up on brightly colored fruits and vegetables will help satisfy your hunger and give your body what it needs to stay healthy. Eat more of the rainbow and fewer starchy white foods.

CHAPTER SIX

Accurate Counting

NUTRITION LABELS

We've already mentioned nutrition labels several times, so let's take a look at an actual label and read through it together. Note that the FDA and food manufacturers are in the process of rolling out a new label with an updated design. This new label will be mandatory by January 2020 for most products, though smaller companies have an additional year to comply. In this chapter, we'll break down the important information presented on both labels and note the differences between them.

The label on page 60 is the version you'll see most often until 2020; the label on page 61 is the updated one. There are three categories of information I always look at first:

1. **Serving Size.** This is the most important. (Remember our discussion of portion size vs. serving size in chapter 4.) On page 60, you'll find this information just under the "Nutrition Facts" title at the top. On page 61, it has moved down a line and the type is in bold and increased in size, so it's easier to spot. In this case, serving size is ⅔ cup or 55g.

2. **Calories.** This number is what to look at next, especially if you are trying to lose weight. Calorie information is the biggest, boldest item on the new label, so it's simple to find. This particular food has 230 calories in ⅔ cup.

3. **Total Carbohydrate.** This is where you get your carb count for this particular food (37g). Total carbs are broken down into Dietary Fiber and Sugars (Total Sugars on the new label). You may see Sugar Alcohol listed here, as well. If you're looking for the best carbs to eat, make sure the sugar count is low and the fiber count is relatively high. (Remember, you want to eat at least 25g of fiber each day.) The new label also distinguishes between naturally occurring sugar and sugar added during the manufacturing process. In our example, one serving of the food contains 12g sugar, 10g of which were added. To calculate the amount of naturally occurring sugar, subtract the Added Sugars from Total Sugars, in this case, 12g to 10g, or 2g.

The next types of information I look for on a nutrition label are:

1. **Total Fat.** You'll see that total fat is broken down into Saturated Fat and Trans Fat. You want the trans fat count to be 0g (see chapter 2 to learn why) and the saturated fat count to be low. The ADA recommends that you restrict your daily

Nutrition Facts

Serving Size 2/3 cup (55g)
Servings Per Container About 8

Amount Per Serving

Calories 230 Calories from Fat 72

% **Daily Value***

Total Fat 8g	**12**%
Saturated Fat 1g	**5**%
Trans Fat 0g	
Cholesterol 0mg	**0**%
Sodium 160mg	**7**%
Total Carbohydrate 37g	**12**%
Dietary Fiber 4g	**16**%
Sugars 12g	
Protein 3g	

Vitamin A	10%
Vitamin C	8%
Calcium	20%
Iron	45%

* Percent Daily Values are based on a 2,000 calorie diet.
Your daily value may be higher or lower depending on
your calorie needs.

	Calories:	2,000	2,500
Total Fat	Less than	65g	80g
Sat Fat	Less than	20g	25g
Cholesterol	Less than	300mg	300mg
Sodium	Less than	2,400mg	2,400mg
Total Carbohydrate		300g	375g
Dietary Fiber		25g	30g

ACCURATE COUNTING

Nutrition Facts

8 servings per container
Serving size   **2/3 cup (55g)**

Amount per serving
Calories   230

	% Daily Value*
Total Fat 8g	**10%**
Saturated Fat 1g	**5%**
Trans Fat 0g	
Cholesterol 0mg	**0%**
Sodium 160mg	**7%**
Total Carbohydrate 37g	**13%**
Dietary Fiber 4g	**14%**
Total Sugars 12g	
Includes 10g Added Sugars	**20%**
Protein 3g	
Vitamin D 2mcg	10%
Calcium 260mg	20%
Iron 8mg	45%
Potassium 235mg	6%

* The % Daily Value (DV) tells you how much a nutrient in a serving of food contributes to a daily diet. 2,000 calories a day is used for general nutrition advice.

ACCURATE COUNTING

saturated fat intake to less than 10 percent of your total daily calories. In our example here, the food contains 1g of saturated fat and 8g of total fat. Sometimes monounsaturated fat and polyunsaturated fat will be listed on a label as well, but this is only required when the manufacturer makes certain claims on their packaging (e.g., "high in monounsaturated fat"). If unsaturated fats aren't listed, you can subtract the saturated and trans fat counts from total fat to get that amount. Our example contains 8 − 1 − 0 = 7g unsaturated fat. Note that "Calories from Fat" will not be included on the new label, because research has shown the amount of fat is actually less important than the type.

2. **Protein.** Here you find the amount of protein contained in the food. If the carb count is relatively high but the protein value is low, you'll probably want to pair it with something high in protein like chicken, fish, or edamame. The food described in this label contains only 3g protein.

3. **Cholesterol.** This shows how much cholesterol is in the food—0mg in this case. If you're watching your cholesterol, keep an eye on this number. This count is also useful if you're trying to follow a totally plant-based diet; if the number reads anything above 0mg, you'll know the food isn't vegan.

4. **Sodium.** The number listed in this category is especially important to people with high blood pressure and/or cardiovascular disease. The sodium recommendation for most people with diabetes is less than 2,300mg per day; those with *hypertension* or heart disease may need to go lower. Keep in mind that processed foods are often particularly high in sodium. In the case of our example, the food contains 160mg of sodium, which is perfectly fine for most people.

You'll find other information on the label, too. Each category contains a "% Daily Value (DV)" to give you a sense of how the food might fit into your overall diet. I don't often pay much attention to these values, as they are calculated assuming you eat 2,000 calories per day, which I personally don't. But I do usually glance at the micronutrient values listed below the protein count. On the new label, however, actual amounts as well as % DV will be required listings for Vitamin D, Calcium, Iron, and Potassium. (Depending on your individual medical profile, these can be useful—if you have kidney disease, for example, knowing the potassium count is particularly important.) Other vitamins and minerals may be listed as well, but are not required.

THE GLYCEMIC INDEX

The glycemic index (GI) measures how quickly foods containing carbs get into your bloodstream as glucose. Foods are ranked on a scale from 1 to 100; a higher ranking means the food will raise your blood sugar more rapidly. Foods ranked 55 or lower are considered to be "low-GI"; those in the 56 to 69 range are "medium-GI"; and those 70 and above are "high-GI." Pure proteins and fats don't receive a GI ranking at all because they don't contain carbs. GI assumes a portion size equal to 50g carbs, which may or may not be reasonable for the particular food at hand.

In contrast to the glycemic index, the glycemic load (GL) takes into account both GI and portion size; basically, you multiply a food's GI by the number of carb grams in a serving and then divide by 100. Foods are considered to be "low GL" if their value is 10 or less. For example, watermelon has a high GI (72), but you'd have to eat a lot of it (4 cups) to get 50g of carbs. Therefore, its GL is relatively low at 4.

See the following chart for the estimated GI and GL values for a few common foods:

FOOD	GI	GL	FOOD	GI	GL
Apple	36	5	Orange juice (unsweetened)	50	12
Banana	48	11	Pear	38	4
Black beans	30	7	Peas	54	4
Blueberries	53	10	Popcorn	65	7
Bread, white	75	11	Potato, white (baked)	85	28
Bread, whole-wheat	69	9	Quinoa	53	13
Carrots	39	2	Raisins	64	28
Cashews	22	3	Raspberries	32	3
Chickpeas	10	3	Rice, brown	50	16
Cola (regular)	63	16	Rice, white	72	29
Cornflakes	81	20	Spaghetti, white	58	26
Glucose	100	50	Spaghetti, whole-grain	42	17
Honey	55	9	Strawberries	40	4
Lentils	28	5	Sugar (sucrose)	68	8
Milk (full-fat or nonfat)	31	4	Sweet potato	70	22
Oatmeal	55	13	Tortilla, corn	52	12
Orange	45	5			

Substituting low-GI foods for high-GI foods may help in controlling your blood sugar. However, the ADA acknowledges that scientific literature on how low-GI foods affect overall blood glucose control is "complex." While some studies have showed low-GI foods to be beneficial, others have not. Most studies up to now have failed to accurately account for fiber, so it's been unclear whether results were related to GI or to fiber content.

Some people manage their diabetes quite well by sticking to a low-GI diet. I eat a lot of fruit and tend to choose low-GI varieties like apples, pears, berries, and citrus most of the time. The ADA recommends carb counting first, and then fine-tuning with GI/GL if desired; personally, I've found that focusing on total carbs and fiber works better for me than just tracking GI and GL. Again, everyone is different, so ask your health care team about whether a low-GI diet might work for you.

IMPROVING ACCURACY

Once you get the hang of the general carb-counting technique, there are several methods you can use to improve your accuracy, save time, and prevent yourself from reinventing the wheel whenever you eat.

Choose recipes with nutrition information. To save yourself some work, stick to cookbooks, websites, and apps that provide nutrition information for each recipe. If there's a recipe you love in a cookbook that doesn't provide carb counts, you can calculate the carbs per serving yourself, and write it down beside the recipe for future reference. Then the next time you make the dish, you won't need to do any calculations. You can also log favorite recipes and their carb counts in apps like MyFitnessPal and Lose It! for easy reference.

Eating out? Plan your meal ahead. If you eat out often at the same places, pull together meal combinations that are compatible with your eating plan. If the restaurant is a chain, you should be able to find nutritional information on their website or through an app. Store the combos in your phone or in a small notebook for quick reference when you're ordering. If you're going somewhere new, consult the restaurant's menu online ahead of time.

Learn how to calculate total carbs vs. net carb counts. Accuracy is particularly important for people who take mealtime insulin. If you are not on insulin, you may be able to simply use total carbs as your count; however, if you take insulin in conjunction with food, you may need to determine your net carb count. Fiber and sugar alcohols don't have much impact on blood glucose, so if you take insulin to cover them, you may suffer a blood sugar low. Subtracting all or some of the fiber and sugar alcohol grams from the total carb count may give you more precise results. Ask your health care team to clarify your particular situation.

Memorize carb counts and portion sizes for go-to meals. If your memory isn't as good as it used to be, keep a list somewhere in your kitchen. You can also log favorite meal combinations in online apps. When you have a good blood sugar day, remember what you ate to include it in a future meal plan. If you use an app, you can email it to yourself or print it.

Pack your lunch. Bring a lunch that meets your needs, and calculate its carb count ahead of time—you may not have the time to do the math when you're at work.

Play "Guess Which Food Has More Carbs." Have everyone come to the dinner table knowing the correct carb counts for two different foods. Each person asks the rest of the group which of their two foods contains more carbs. If I were playing, I might use 1 cup of pea soup versus a grilled cheese sandwich on white bread. Folks might be surprised to learn that the grilled cheese has fewer carbs (40g) than the soup (56g)!

Stick to the same brands. Use the same brands of food products consistently, and familiarize yourself with their carb counts. A serving of one brand of yogurt, for example, may have more or fewer carbs than another brand. If you always buy the same brand, you won't have to keep reading the label.

Weigh your food. To improve your accuracy when counting carbs, weigh your food. For example, CalorieKing says that one medium pear has about 28g of carbs. But it also notes that "medium" means 7 ounces. If you weigh the pear you're about to eat and it comes in at 5 ounces, that's only 20g ($5 \div 7 = 0.71$, $0.71 \times 28 = 19.88$, round to 20).

HANDY MATH

Sometimes the math involved in carb counting can feel overwhelming. Here are a few shortcuts to help you estimate carb counts:

- **Carb units:** You may find it easier to think of foods as carb units instead of grams. In chapter 4, the serving sizes listed for common high-carb foods all contain roughly 15g of carbs (e.g., ⅓ cup rice), so you might consider 15g of carbs as one unit. Therefore, if you calculated your appropriate amount of carbs per meal to be 45g, you could think of it instead as 3 units of 15g each. You'd know you could eat a Mexican side dish featuring ⅔ cup black beans plus ⅓ cup brown rice, and you'd be close to your target of 45g of carbs without having to count.

- **Combination foods:** Determining how to count combination foods can be tricky, especially if you don't know exactly what's in them. Dishes falling into this category include casseroles, soups, and stews containing both starches and vegetables (e.g., chicken pot pie). The rule of thumb is to count 1 cup as 30g of carbs. (Remember that 1 cup is about the size of your fist.) If it's a broth-based soup featuring mainly protein and nonstarchy vegetables, 1 cup is roughly 15g of carbs.

- **"Free" foods:** You may be able to treat nonstarchy vegetables as "free" foods, meaning you may not need to count their carbs at all. Experiment to see how these foods affect your blood sugar, then decide whether or not you need to count them.

CHAPTER SEVEN

Meal Planning

MEAL PLANNING WORKS

If you shop for groceries when you're starving or don't take a list, do you buy foods you really shouldn't be eating? Trying to manage your diabetes without a meal plan is similar in this way: You eat more carbs than you should, they aren't the best types of carbs you could choose, your blood sugar (and weight) inevitably goes up, and you become frustrated. Instead, if you did a little bit of planning, you'd know when to eat, what to eat, and how much to eat each day. Your confidence in managing your diabetes would grow, and it would be much easier to stay on track.

I know what you're thinking: *But I don't have time to plan my meals*. Trust me, it's worth it to make time. Once you get a few plans under your belt, you can use them over and over again. And your blood sugar will thank you.

Although meal planning requires some work up front, its benefits are definitely worth it. Consider the following advantages:

- **Balanced meals.** Your meals will have the right balance of carbs, protein, and fat.
- **Calories on target.** Your daily calorie intake will be the right amount.
- **Carbs spread throughout the day.** Your daily carb allowance will be spread out to better control your blood sugar.
- **Less thinking.** You won't have to come up with new ideas every day at mealtime.
- **Minimized stress.** Life will ultimately be less stressful. (In chapter 9, we'll learn about the impact of stress on diabetes management.)
- **Nutritious food.** You'll eat healthy foods you've planned in advance.
- **Shared cooking.** Other members of your household can help cook when they know the plan.
- **Simplified shopping.** Grocery shopping will be easier.

BASICS

This may sound like a dream come true, but where do you start? How do you develop one of these magic meal plans?

One problem I have when I sit down to plan is that there are just too many options available. If you're like me, you own a ton of cookbooks, you subscribe to several food magazines, and you drool over lots of recipes online. Okay, maybe you aren't like me. But the number of choices you have when deciding what to cook can be overwhelming. The following are some approaches I use to make the process less daunting.

Cook with the Seasons

Focusing your meals on seasonal ingredients helps both your diet and your budget. In-season produce tastes better and costs less, especially if it's locally grown. I keep five folders in my kitchen marked "Spring," "Summer," "Fall," "Winter," and "Anytime." So if I come across an asparagus recipe I want to try, it goes in the "Spring" folder. Then when I sit down to meal plan in March, I pull out the "Spring" folder and immediately become inspired.

Pick a Nightly Dinner Theme

When you're getting started with meal planning, it can be really helpful to have a theme for each night's dinner that's consistent from week to week. For example:

- **Monday** is vegetarian (you've heard of Meatless Monday, right?)
- **Tuesday** is Mexican (in the spirit of Taco Tuesday)
- **Wednesday** is Asian
- **Thursday** is Italian
- **Friday** is fish
- **Saturday** is Indian
- **Sunday** is comfort food

Switch up the themes to suit your family. If your crew isn't into international foods, pick a specific protein for each night (e.g., Thursday is chicken night). Assigning nightly themes helps narrow your options when you plan your dinners for the week. You might even ask other family members to come up with menu ideas that fit the themes.

Have a Few Go-to Breakfasts

Come up with a few go-to breakfasts that work for you. We have five or six that we eat on rotation throughout the busy work week, and then we try to make something a little more creative on the weekends. Sometimes we concoct a breakfast casserole or crustless quiche on Sunday, and reheat leftovers on Monday and Tuesday. Our go-to breakfasts of the moment include scrambled eggs with salsa and avocado, cottage cheese pancakes with blueberries, high-protein smoothies, overnight oats with apples and walnuts, chia pudding with raspberries and pumpkin seeds, and hard-boiled eggs with whole-grain toast and fruit. If you need breakfasts to be portable, keep that in mind when you plan.

Easy Lunch Options

When you think about lunch options for your meal plan, consider soups, stews, salads, and leftovers. Make a big pot of vegetable-heavy soup or stew on the weekend, and portion it into appropriate containers to eat for lunch during the week. Salads featuring lots of raw vegetables topped with lean protein and a homemade vinaigrette work well, too. My very favorite lunch is leftover anything (assuming the original was good, of course). Most recipes I make serve four; even though there are only two of us in the house, I always make full recipes and count on the leftovers for another meal.

Chart It Out

Use some sort of chart to map everything out. You can fit a less detailed view for the entire week on one page, or you can opt for a more detailed plan for each day. (See sample charts later in this chapter.) For each meal, make sure you have some protein and fat, plus your recommended amounts of calories and carbs. You can plan meals only in this format, or you can add a row or two to the chart to cover snacks, as well. If you don't want to work too hard at this, type "diabetes meal plans" into Google or another search engine to get ideas.

TIPS AND TRICKS

Now that you know the basics of meal planning, let's talk about a few ways to streamline the process:

Chop vegetables on your prep day. Carrots, celery, bell peppers, broccoli, cauliflower, and cucumbers can be used in salads or as snacks during the week. If several recipes requiring diced onions are in your plan, chop as much as you'll need ahead of time.

Factor leftovers into your plan. Why cook more than once when you don't have to? Make twice the amount of a recipe you need for a single meal, and then eat the leftovers later in the week.

Pick one or two prep days during the week. If you work Monday through Friday and have weekends off, pick Saturday or Sunday. Make a casserole, soup, or stew, portion it appropriately, and refrigerate (if you'll eat it soon) or freeze. Whisk together a home-made salad dressing that will last your family all week. Chop vegetables and make a dip (see page 74).

Plan around calendar items. When pulling together your plan, take a look at your calendar for the upcoming week. If you'll be racing from work straight to a soccer game and won't get home until 8 p.m. on Thursday, you may need to factor in a restaurant meal or leftovers you can quickly heat up when you get home.

Post your meal plan. If everyone in the household knows the plan, they can pitch in to help cook, and you won't be asked, "What's for dinner?" ad nauseam. When I post our plan on the refrigerator door, I'm often pleasantly surprised that, if I'm working late, my husband will start cooking when he gets hungry.

Think ahead to the next day's meal. Is there anything you can do today to make life easier tomorrow? For example, if it's Tuesday, and you plan to grill chicken breasts on Wednesday, place your frozen chicken in the refrigerator overnight to thaw.

Whip up a healthy dip. Homemade guacamole or hummus will taste great with your prechopped vegetables when you need a snack. Always have at least one healthy dip option in your refrigerator.

MEAL PLANNER

There are many ways to map out your meal plan. If you want to be able to see the entire week at a glance and fit the entire meal plan on one page, then it won't contain as much detail. Alternatively, if you prefer a higher level of tracking and logging for each meal, use a daily plan; in this case you'll need seven pages for the week.

Weekly Plan

The template on page 76 shows one way to lay out a weekly plan. Feel free to tailor it to meet your needs. If you want to include a snack, add a row. If you don't care about nightly themes, just delete them. An actual weekly plan might look like the one on page 78.

Daily Plan

Page 80 shows one possibility for mapping out a more-detailed daily plan. If you go this route, I recommend using spreadsheet software like Microsoft® Excel or Apple® Numbers so the calculations will be done for you automatically. You could also add a column for pre-meal or post-meal BG, if desired. If you take insulin, you may want to add a way to track your dosages in conjunction with your meals.

An actual daily plan might look like the chart on page 82. While the daily plan contains a lot of useful information, it is more difficult to pull together than a high-level weekly plan. Note that nutritional information for each item in the sample chart was obtained from CalorieKing, MyFitnessPal, or Lose It! and should be considered an estimate only. If you need exact carb counts for insulin dosing purposes, please do the calculations yourself.

I recommend starting with the less detailed weekly plan and logging everything in an app or using an online tool when you eat. Then you can just print (or email) your daily diary that includes the additional detail. All the work will be done for you, and you can reuse the daily plan in the future.

WEEK OF: DAILY CALORIES:

	MONDAY	TUESDAY	WEDNESDAY
BREAKFAST TARGET CARBS: 45G			
LUNCH TARGET CARBS: 45G			
THEME			
DINNER TARGET CARBS: 45G			
DO-AHEAD PREP			

THURSDAY	FRIDAY	SATURDAY	SUNDAY

*Downloadable template available at diabeticfoodie.com.

	MONDAY	**TUESDAY**	**WEDNESDAY**
BREAKFAST **TARGET CARBS:** **45G**	Spinach Smoothie with Apples & Grapes* Boiled Egg	Cottage Cheese Pancakes Fresh Strawberries Turkey Bacon	Cottage Cheese Pancakes Frozen Blueberries (thawed)
LUNCH **TARGET CARBS:** **45G**	Turkey Barley Vegetable Soup* Edamame (in the pod)	Turkey Barley Vegetable Soup* Clementines	Leftover Chicken Enchilada–Stuffed Acorn Squash Pear
THEME	Vegetarian	Mexican	Asian
DINNER **TARGET CARBS:** **45G**	Greek Salad with Tomatoes, Cucumbers, Chickpeas, Mozzarella Crackers (e.g., Nut-Thins)	Chicken Enchilada–Stuffed Acorn Squash* Steamed Broccoli	Scallop Stir-Fry with Bok Choy & Carrots Brown Rice Egg-Drop Soup
DO-AHEAD PREP	Make cottage cheese pancakes to reheat for breakfast on Tues. and Wed.	Cook enough turkey bacon for Thurs. salad, chop veggies for Wed. stir-fry	Precook chicken for Thurs. pizza, make enough rice for Sat. dinner

THURSDAY	FRIDAY	SATURDAY	SUNDAY
Scrambled Eggs with Salsa & Cheese Avocado Toast (on whole-grain bread) Banana	Chia Pudding with Raspberries, Almonds, Pumpkin Seeds	Quinoa & Oatmeal Blend with Almond Milk, Walnuts, Pumpkin Seeds Canadian Bacon	Turkey Sausage Casserole with Veggie Tots* Whole-Grain Toast Orange Wedges
Restaurant meal: Small Turkey Sub (on whole-grain roll) Dill Pickle Spear	Leftover Cauliflower Crust Pizza Apple	Roasted Red Pepper Soup with Shrimp Tossed Salad	Leftover Grilled Salmon Spinach Salad with Beets, Goat Cheese Blueberries
Italian	Fish	Indian	Comfort
Cauliflower Crust Pizza* topped with Chicken & Sun-Dried Tomatoes Spinach Salad with Turkey Bacon & Apple	Grilled Salmon Sautéed Brussels Sprouts Baked Sweet Potato	Spinach Curry (Palak Paneer)* Brown Rice Sliced Mango	Chicken Chili Verde with Hominy & Pumpkin* Clementines
Trim Brussels sprouts and cut in half for Fri. dinner	Peel and devein shrimp for Sat. soup	Roast beets for Sun. salad	Chop vegetables and make salad dressing and/or soup for next week

*Recipe available at diabeticfoodie.com

DATE:

BREAKFAST

LUNCH

MEAL PLANNING

DINNER

TOTAL NUMBERS

TARGET NUMBERS

CALORIES	CARBS (G)	PROTEIN (G)	FAT (G)	FIBER (G)	SODIUM (MG)
CALORIES	CARBS (G)	PROTEIN (G)	FAT (G)	FIBER (G)	SODIUM (MG)

DATE:

BREAKFAST

Cottage Cheese Pancakes – 1 serving

Fresh Raspberries – ¾ cup

Turkey Bacon – 2 slices

MEAL PLANNING

LUNCH

Turkey Barley Vegetable Soup* – 2 cups

Clementines – 2

DINNER

Chicken Enchilada–Stuffed Acorn Squash – 1 serving

Broccoli (steamed) – 1 cup

Apple (sliced) – 1 medium

TOTAL NUMBERS

TARGET NUMBERS

CALORIES	CARBS (G)	PROTEIN (G)	FAT (G)	FIBER (G)	SODIUM (MG)
315	21	24	12	3	431
48	11	1	1	6	1
70	0	4	5	0	280
226	20	19	8	4	716
70	18	1	0	3	1
440	32	35	20	5	748
30	6	3	0	2	29
93	25	1	0	4	2
1,292	133	88	46	27	2,208
1,300	130			> 25	< 2,300
CALORIES	CARBS (G)	PROTEIN (G)	FAT (G)	FIBER (G)	SODIUM (MG)

CHAPTER EIGHT

Tracking Yourself

TRACKING TOOLS

Tracking is key to making the carb-counting process work. If you don't track, you won't be able to analyze your results and make adjustments that can help you control your blood sugar more successfully. By tracking, for example, I've learned that my fasting BG numbers are much better when I eat an early dinner and a handful of nuts before I go to bed. Sadly, I've also learned that pizza is a food I should not eat very often. If I crave pizza now, I have one small slice plus a big salad instead of two or three slices. But that's a positive adjustment I made based on my data. And I still get to eat pizza.

What's the best way to track? It all depends on how you like to do things. You can go old-school with a classic calendar or notebook, or you can log everything electronically. You can also use a combination. Here are a few options for you to try:

Apps or online tools: Use one of the apps or online tools mentioned in chapter 2. An added benefit of using an app is that you can easily see the percentages of your calories coming from carbs, fat, and protein at any point during the day. If you eat more carbs than you planned at lunch, you can make adjustments at dinner to keep your daily total in range.

Meal-planning tools like dinner themes or seasonal ingredients: Utilize one of the meal planning tools in chapter 7. If you eat what's in your plan, the tracking is already done.

Old-fashioned food diary: Keep a food diary. Write down what you eat at every meal, along with each item's carb count. If you're trying to lose (or gain) weight, write down calories, too. You can even jot down what your BG was two hours after each meal.

Spreadsheet: Track everything in a spreadsheet. Just like the apps, it will do the math for you.

BE HONEST

To avoid unnecessary complications, here are a few ways to help keep yourself honest:

Don't tell your CDE/RD you will make changes that aren't realistic for you. For example, don't agree to cut out all fast food if you are frequently on the road and eat it often. Instead, work with your health care team to figure out how to make better choices when you do eat fast food.

Make sure you are accurately documenting portion sizes. Maybe you're honestly logging the amount of carbs you *think* a particular food contains, but you're actually eating twice that amount. Measure and then look up the food so you'll *know*.

Stop thinking of your BG readings as "good" or "bad." They aren't judgments; they're just data points. You are either "in range" or you aren't. If you aren't, don't beat yourself up; just make adjustments so that you are.

PART III

Healthy Lifestyle

Watching your carb intake is important, but successfully managing your diabetes also requires that you maintain a healthy lifestyle. You need to manage stress, make good food choices when you're away from home, and be physically active every day. Need incentive to exercise? A small study of *Biggest Loser* contestants showed that, while diet may help you lose weight initially, it's exercise that helps you keep it off. Exercise also helps improve your sleep and manage stress.

Chapter 9 will take a look at the importance of exercise and provide some tips on how to fit physical activity into your day. You'll also discover why it's important to monitor your heart health, get adequate sleep, and control the stress in your life.

Chapter 10 will explain why cooking at home is best for monitoring your blood sugar, and offer simple ways to make grocery shopping less of a chore. You'll also find strategies for staying on track when you eat out and how to snack in a healthy way.

Finally, chapter 11 will summarize the main concepts you've learned in the book and provide 10 must-do tips to help you count carbs and stay healthy. To conclude, you'll find out why support from friends, family, coworkers, the diabetes online community, support groups, conferences, and medical professionals is so crucial to your diabetes management success.

CHAPTER NINE

Your Health Goals

EXERCISE WORKS

Whether or not you have diabetes, exercise is one of the most important things you can do to stay healthy. Physical activity increases your body's sensitivity to insulin, which means you won't need as much, since the insulin you have can do more work. One effect is that you have more energy. Exercise also strengthens your heart, improves the quality of your sleep, and helps you more successfully manage the stress in your life. But you probably know this already. So why don't you exercise regularly?

Being physically active doesn't require a gym membership, expensive equipment, or trendy athletic wear. But by all means, invest in those things if they motivate you. Increasing your physical activity simply requires commitment.

The ADA recommends 150 minutes of exercise each week, ideally getting some in each day. This is especially important for people with type 2 diabetes and prediabetes. A combination of cardio exercise (walking, running, aerobics, etc.) plus resistance training (exercise bands, dumbbells, weight machines, etc.) appears to be most effective. The ADA also recommends getting up and moving around every 30 minutes if you sit for prolonged periods of time during the day.

Incorporating physical activity into your daily schedule doesn't have to be a grind. Here are a few easy ways to get yourself moving:

Do yardwork. Gardening, shoveling snow, mowing the grass, and raking leaves all count as exercise. You even get a nutritional bonus: Spending time outdoors will give you a boost of vitamin D (the "sunshine vitamin").

Move during the workday. If your job is sedentary, set a timer for 25 minutes each time you sit down. When it goes off, get up and move around for 5 minutes—stretch, do yoga poses, or simply march in place. It doesn't matter what you do, just move your body.

Use exercise videos. I discovered these about a year ago, and they have truly changed my life. I don't have to worry about the weather, and I can do any type of exercise I want, anytime I feel like doing it. Aerobics, yoga, and resistance training with dumbbells are my favorites. Check out the videos offered by DiabetesStrong (diabetesstrong.com)—they were created by a personal trainer who just happens to have type 1 diabetes.

Take walks. This can be for as little as 10 minutes after each meal, or for a longer period whenever possible during the day. Take the dog, walk with a friend or family member, enjoy nature, or listen to a podcast or music.

HEART HEALTH

Living with diabetes greatly increases your chances of suffering a heart attack or stroke and actually doubles the risk of death from one of these conditions. Why is that? Recall from chapter 1 that glucose is "sticky" and binds to proteins in your blood vessels. If one has chronically high blood sugar levels, this can lead to blood vessel damage, a major contributor to heart disease and stroke.

Fortunately, there are several things you can do to keep your heart healthy:

Exercise. Start slow and increase your intensity over time. Your heart is a muscle that gets stronger when you exercise, just like your other muscles do.

Keep your BG in range. Better blood sugar control leads to healthier blood vessels and a healthier heart.

Maintain a healthy weight. Being overweight can increase your risk for heart attack and stroke. Even if you're not overweight, excess belly fat can increase your risk, too.

Monitor your ABCs. A is for *A1C*, B is for blood pressure, and C is for cholesterol. Target numbers and frequency of testing will vary, depending on your particular case, so check with your health care team to see what's right for you. In the meantime, here is some basic information to keep in mind:

A1C: The A1C test measures your average blood sugar over the last three months. The A1C goal for most people with diabetes is less than 7 percent. Have your A1C tested every 3 to 6 months.

Blood pressure: Check your blood pressure every time you visit the doctor and regularly at home, too, if you've been diagnosed with hypertension. Healthy blood pressure is 120/80 mmHg; if you have both diabetes and hypertension, your goal is below 140/90 mmHg.

Cholesterol: Both cholesterol and triglycerides are *lipids*, fat-like substances found in your blood. There are two primary types of cholesterol: *low-density lipoprotein (LDL)*, the "bad" stuff, and *high-density lipoprotein (HDL)*, the "good stuff." Aim for LDL less than 100 mg/dL and HDL greater than 40 mg/dL (women) and greater than 50 mg/dL (men). Triglycerides should be less than 150 mg/dL. Have your lipids tested once a year or so.

Quit smoking. Smoking damages your blood vessels, too, so smoking with diabetes is a double whammy.

SLEEP ESSENTIALS

Do you get enough sleep? I'm guessing you probably don't. In the United States, we are so sleep-deprived that entire books have been written on the subject. What is *enough*, anyway? The National Sleep Foundation recommends that adults under the age of 64 get about 7 to 9 hours each night and adults 65 or older get 7 to 8 hours. A small study on Japanese adults with type 2 diabetes indicated that the optimal range was 6.5 to 7.4 hours per night. Results showed that both too much sleep and too little had negative effects on blood glucose levels. Aiming for 7 hours of sleep nightly seems to be a good goal.

If insomnia is preventing you from getting the sleep you need, try these strategies for improving both the quantity and quality of your sleep:

Avoid overeating or not eating enough. Don't go to bed either extremely hungry or miserably full.

Be comfortable in bed. Make sure your bed, pillow, and sheets are cozy and inviting.

Create conducive sleeping conditions. Keep your bedroom dark, quiet, and cool.

Establish a calming ritual. Ease into a relaxing bedtime routine; for example, take a bath or write in a journal.

Exercise regularly. Set aside some time to work out on a consistent basis.

Quiet your thoughts. Meditate just before you go to sleep. Try apps such as Buddhify or Headspace.

Shut down electronic devices. Turn off all screens (TVs, computers, phones, tablets, etc.) within an hour of bedtime.

Stick to a consistent bedtime. Make an effort to maintain the same sleeping schedule, even on weekends.

DON'T STRESS

When your body is under stress, whether it's due to an actual physical threat or something purely emotional, your liver pumps out extra glucose as additional energy to deal with the situation at hand. This works fine in people who don't have diabetes. Unfortunately, for those of us who do, our bodies don't always have enough insulin available to shuttle this extra glucose where it's needed, so it builds up in our bloodstream. The result is a prolonged state of elevated blood sugar.

This may be okay for infrequent, short-term plights. But if the stress in your life is constant, finding ways to manage it is critical for improving your diabetes control. So how do you achieve this? Try following these tips to cut down your daily stress:

Allow plenty of time. Avoid the panic of running late. Then when you're heading to an appointment, you won't need to rush.

Breathe deeply. When you feel anxious, take a moment for a long, calming breath.

Communicate effectively. Don't let sticky situations fester.

Exercise regularly. (Are you convinced yet?)

Get a pet. Dogs and cats are known to have a soothing effect on their owners.

Get enough sleep. See page 91 for tips on improving sleep.

Identify what's stressing you, and brainstorm ways to better manage it. For example, if money is a problem, you might use a service like Mint.com to start logging your expenses in an effort to understand exactly where your money is going; once the situation is clear, you can work out strategies for spending less. (Data tracking to the rescue again.)

Increase your social interactions. Take your mind off personal concerns and engage with others.

Keep a journal. Writing down your thoughts can bring clarity.

Learn something new. Acquire a skill, or take on a new hobby.

Meditate or schedule quiet time each day. Even five minutes will help.

Share the burden of household tasks. Why go it alone?

Stop being a perfectionist. You don't need the added pressure.

Stretch daily or do yoga. Bring relief to your body, and it will also spread to your mind.

CHAPTER TEN

Out and About

GROCERY SHOPPING

Is grocery shopping the household chore you dread the most? After all, it requires planning your meals, making a list, driving to the store, getting frustrated when you can't find the items you want, dodging people who have no business operating a shopping cart, spending a lot of money, and lugging heavy bags. What's to like? It's no surprise that people are cooking less and eating in restaurants more and more.

Despite the coordination and prep time required, cooking at home is one of the best ways to eat healthy. Preparing your own food allows you to easily control the quality of carbs, types of fat, and amount of sodium in your diet, among other factors. So what if I told you there are ways to make grocery shopping a little less burdensome? Would you be more likely to cook at home?

Here are a few strategies for streamlining your grocery shopping experience and choosing healthy foods:

Always have a list in hand. Only shop when you have a list and you aren't feeling rushed or stressed. Don't try it when you're hungry or have kids in tow. You'll be way too tempted to throw things in the cart without paying attention to the quality of your choices.

Buy frozen and canned fruits and vegetables. These can be perfectly healthy and will keep longer than their fresh counterparts. Just look for brands with no added sugar and minimal sodium.

Check out bulk foods. Become familiar with the bulk food aisle. It's a great place to stock up on nuts, seeds, and high-fiber grains.

Focus on produce, proteins, and dairy products. In other words, avoid the center aisles of the store that are overflowing with processed foods.

Let someone else shop. Ask someone else in the household to do the shopping—they might actually enjoy it.

Order groceries online. Once you've placed your order, either pick them up yourself or have them delivered. By ordering in advance, you'll be much more likely to stick to your list.

Seek out farmers' markets. Buy as much of your produce as possible at farmers' markets. Purchasing directly from growers means you get the freshest possible fruits and vegetables—often items for sale were just picked that morning. Shopping at farmers' markets will also reduce the time you spend at the grocery store.

EATING OUT

No matter how good your intentions or how well you've laid out your meal plans, you can't avoid it—there will be times when you eat out. For some of us, it happens quite often. If I'm ever visiting a new town, you can bet I'll be checking out interesting places that serve local specialties. And while it's easier to eat healthily when you cook your own meals, you can still eat restaurant food and manage to stay on-track in terms of counting carbs.

Here's how you can stick to your diet while eating in restaurants or ordering takeout:

1. **Check the menu before you go.** Search for dishes that fit your meal plan, then decide ahead of time what you will order. You can even pre-enter your choices into your food diary as a reminder.

2. **Select a restaurant that serves small plates.** Ordering a selection of small plates (a.k.a. tapas) allows for better portion control and variety.

3. **Request low-carb options in advance.** If you're going to a fine dining establishment where the menu changes daily, let them know when you make the reservation that you have diabetes and would appreciate low-carb options the night you plan to be there. Good chefs will appreciate the challenge as long as you give them enough notice.

4. **Just say no to the bread basket.** Decline the basket full of bread—that goes for chips, too.

5. **Choose an appetizer rather than a full-sized entrée.** A starter like steamed shrimp or mussels plus a side salad or bowl of vegetable soup makes a great meal.

6. **Order a simple protein with a side of vegetables.** This is always a healthier option than "mixed" dishes like casseroles; plus, this will allow you to follow the plate method (see page 55). If your meal arrives and the protein or starch takes up more than one-quarter of the plate, take a portion of an appropriate serving size, and immediately place the rest in a to-go container. And make sure at least one of your vegetables is green.

7. **Don't order items you'd avoid at home.** You normally steer clear of fried foods, "white" foods, and sweetened beverages, so don't order them just because you're eating out.

8. **Ask for substitutions.** This is an easy one. For example, can you get steamed broccoli instead of potatoes?

9. **Have a big salad topped with protein.** You've got lots of options here. You might choose grilled chicken, shrimp, or fish, and you may have a choice of greens as well. If so, go with spinach or another dark leafy green instead of iceberg lettuce.

10. **Split a main course.** Main courses tend to be huge, so share an entrée with someone and order a side salad.

11. **Keep your salad dressing simple.** If you order any type of salad, choose a vinaigrette or stick to just oil and vinegar. Balsamic vinegar by itself makes a sweet, zesty salad dressing, too.

12. **Resist the dessert temptation.** Instead, order a cup of herbal tea or black coffee, and if you like, ask for a serving of fresh fruit.

SNACK SMART

"What can I eat as a snack?" is a question I hear frequently. Folks who munch on chips, crackers, and candy need lower carb options once they are diagnosed with diabetes. Before I was diagnosed, my daily 3 p.m. ritual was to visit the vending machine at work and get a regular Coke® and a bag of M&M'S®. I don't recommend this type of snacking.

Fortunately, there are many tasty snacks that will keep you from straying off your meal plan. In general, the best snacks include a balance of carbs, protein, and fat. Here are a few of my favorites:

OUT AND ABOUT

Energy bites: Homemade no-bake energy bites are easy to prepare and usually involve dates, nuts, seeds, coconut, and spices like cinnamon. Basically, you pulse everything in a food processor and then roll it into small balls. I especially like energy bites as a post-workout snack.

Fruit plus walnuts or string cheese: Apple chunks or pear slices combined with some protein and fat like nuts, cheese, or nut butter make a perfectly balanced snack.

Gorp (or trail mix): I make my own and portion it into snack-size plastic zippered bags. I keep a bag in my purse and take several whenever I'm going on a trip. Prepackaged trail mix usually includes a lot of dried fruit and sweetened granola, so I avoid it. Instead, my version often contains walnuts, almonds, cashews, pumpkin seeds, and a few dark chocolate chips (though I skip the chocolate during warmer weather because it melts and makes a mess). Sometimes I add unsweetened coconut chips or a tiny bit of dried fruit.

Homemade dip and raw vegetables: We pre-chop celery and carrot sticks and always try to keep some healthy dip like guacamole, hummus, or salsa in our refrigerator. One of our favorite Super Bowl snacks is Nacho Celery Sticks—celery topped with a mixture of salsa and guacamole, then sprinkled with cheddar cheese. We also like to experiment with different flavors of hummus—a few we've enjoyed include Buffalo wing, artichoke, white bean, and edamame.

Plain Greek yogurt (or cottage cheese) with berries: Greek yogurt has fewer carbs and more protein than regular yogurt, so it's a good choice for people with diabetes. Most berries, especially raspberries and strawberries, are low-GI foods and make great toppings. For additional flavor, sprinkle the yogurt with ground cinnamon and your favorite nuts and seeds, if desired. If you aren't a yogurt fan, cottage cheese works well, too.

CHAPTER ELEVEN

Staying on Track

10 TIPS

We've covered a lot of territory in this book, from the science of blood sugar to how to handle stress. While it's all important, it can be a lot of information to take in all at once. If you feel overwhelmed, just focus on the guiding principles that follow—even if you disregard everything else. Following these 10 tips faithfully (and honestly)—with both commitment and perseverance—will improve your diet, blood sugar control, and overall health.

1. **Strive for a balance of carbs and other nutrients.** Have a general idea of how many carbs you should eat daily. Spread them throughout the day as you plan your meals and snacks. Strive for a balance of carbs, protein, and fat each time you eat.

2. **Track the numbers and effects.** Track how many carbs you eat and how each meal/snack affects your BG. You can do this on paper, online, or via an app. Just do it.

3. **Favor carbs that are rich in both fiber and nutrients.** Avoid starchy white foods and sugar. Eat lots of colorful vegetables and fruits.

4. **Cook at home as often as possible.** This will ensure the most effective control over your diet. Get everyone in your household involved to make eating at home less of a burden.

5. **Read nutrition labels.** Also look up fresh foods in apps or online databases, so you'll know exact carb counts. Don't guess.

6. **Maintain a healthy lifestyle.** This includes exercising regularly, getting enough sleep, and managing stress. Visit members of your health care team several times a year to make sure you're on the right track.

7. **Control your portion sizes.** Customize the amounts you eat of different foods based on your individual carb allowance.

8. **Choose lean proteins.** These include proteins like poultry, shellfish, and tofu, but also try to eat fatty fish once or twice a week.

9. **Consume mostly unsaturated fats.** Make olive oil your go-to cooking fat.

10. **Experiment to find what works for you.** Only with trial and error will you know what truly works best for you. Since everyone is different, there is no one-size-fits-all "diabetes diet." Review data you collect via your tracking process, and use it to fine-tune your meal plans. And don't beat yourself up if you fall off the wagon—the important thing is that you get back on and move forward.

WITH A LITTLE HELP

Managing diabetes on your own can be overwhelming. Fortunately, many resources are available to assist you. The critical thing to remember is *don't be afraid to ask for help*. Needing assistance doesn't mean you're weak; it means you're human.

Here are some places to find support when you need it:

CDEs and RDs: If counting carbs, dosing mealtime insulin appropriately, and figuring out the best foods to eat are tasks that overwhelm you, consult a CDE or RD. Their expert guidance will make things easier to manage.

Diabetes classes: Many hospitals and local health departments offer diabetes education courses. Ask your doctor, CDE, or RD what might be available in your area. The YMCA also offers two types of diabetes programs in some locations: one benefits people with prediabetes, and the other is for people who have been diagnosed with type 2.

Diabetes conferences: Attending a diabetes conference will truly open your eyes. If you have one type of diabetes, you'll learn about the other types. You'll also meet other people struggling with the same issues you are, and you'll get to hear speakers with a wealth of knowledge and great tips. Conferences and seminars for people with diabetes are frequently held in various locations by Taking Control of Your Diabetes (TCOYD), DiabetesSisters, the Diabetes UnConference, and other organizations.

Diabetic Foodie: My website, diabeticfoodie.com, offers diabetic-friendly recipes and healthy eating tips. Feel free to contact me with questions or comments about carb counting, diet, or any specific challenges you're facing. I'll help if I can. I'd love to hear from you on social media or via email (info@diabeticfoodie.com).

Diabetes online community (DOC): Websites such as TuDiabetes (tudiabetes.org), Diabetes Daily (diabetesdaily.com), dLife (dlife.

com), Diabetes Mine (healthline.com/diabetesmine), and diaTribe (diatribe.org) offer a wealth of information and online forums for people with diabetes. There are also frequent Twitter chats, Facebook Live events, and other ways to connect via social media.

Diabetes-related events: Organizations like the ADA and the Juvenile Diabetes Research Foundation (JDRF) sponsor events such as bike races, walks, and marathons to raise money for diabetes research. Even if you aren't an athlete, you can volunteer at these events and meet a lot of diabetes advocates.

Friends, family, and coworkers: Tell them you have diabetes and explain what that means for your lifestyle. Make sure they understand what foods are best for your diet. I once heard Ina Garten (Barefoot Contessa) say that when she throws a dinner party, instead of inquiring about food allergies or dietary restrictions, she simply asks her guests what they don't eat. She said the reason they don't eat particular foods doesn't matter to her menu planning and simply isn't any of her business. So just tell the people in your life what you don't eat.

Support groups: Over the years, I've belonged to several support groups, and all of them have helped keep me on track. People coping with the same issues you face just "get it," no explanation required. Check to see if your county's board of health or a local hospital offers a diabetes support group. I also highly recommend DiabetesSisters (diabetessisters.org) for women aged 18 or older. (Disclaimer: I am a DiabetesSisters group leader.)

Glossary

A1C: *See* hemoglobin A1C

acanthosis nigricans: Dark spots on the skin, especially at the back of the neck, in folds of skin, or in the groin area that may be symptoms of insulin resistance

alpha-linolenic acid (ALA): An omega-3 essential fatty acid

amino acids: Substances obtained from protein you eat or generated in your body to perform certain functions like repairing muscle tissue

antioxidant: A substance found in food that protects the body from the negative effects of harmful molecules known as free radicals

beta-carotene: A substance found in naturally orange and yellow foods that is converted to vitamin A in the body

beta cells: The cells in the pancreas responsible for producing insulin

biguanides: A class of type 2 diabetes medications that make your body tissues more sensitive to insulin and lower the amount of glucose produced by the liver (e.g., metformin)

blood glucose (BG): The amount of glucose present in the bloodstream (a.k.a. blood sugar)

carbohydrate: A macronutrient found in foods like vegetables, fruits, grains, dairy products, and desserts

celiac disease: An autoimmune disease triggered by eating gluten (wheat), which may result in a severely damaged small intestine

certified diabetes educator (CDE): A health care provider who has had comprehensive training in prediabetes, diabetes prevention, and diabetes management

cholesterol: A waxy fat-like substance found in the blood used by your body to make hormones and vitamins

dawn phenomenon (dawn effect): Early-morning high blood glucose triggered by the body's release of hormones

diabetic neuropathy: Nerve damage caused by diabetes that may result in tingling, numbness, or pain in the feet, legs, hands, or arms

diabetic retinopathy: A type of vision impairment that occurs when chronically elevated blood glucose damages the blood vessels in the eyes

dipeptidyl peptidase-4 (DPP-4): An enzyme that removes incretins from the body

dipeptidyl peptidase-4 (DPP-4) inhibitors: A class of type 2 diabetes medications that block the action of DPP-4 in the body and allow incretins to do their job (e.g., Januvia®)

docosahexaenoic acid (DHA): An omega-3 fatty acid that can be made in the body, but is better obtained from foods like fatty fish

eicosapentaenoic acid (EPA): An omega-3 fatty acid that can be made in the body, but is better obtained from foods like fatty fish

enzymes: Proteins that speed up certain biochemical reactions in the body, like breaking down starch during digestion

essential amino acid: An amino acid that cannot be generated by your body and must be obtained from food

essential fatty acid (EFA): A fatty acid that cannot be manufactured by the body and must be obtained from food

fat: A macronutrient found in foods like oils, butter, avocado, and fatty fish, which supplies energy to your body and protects your vital organs

fiber: A complex carbohydrate, also known as "roughage," that has little effect on blood sugar

fructose: A type of sugar found in foods like fruit and honey that is metabolized directly by the liver

gastrointestinal (GI) tract: The part of the body's digestive system that includes the esophagus, stomach, and intestines

gestational diabetes: A condition where a pregnant woman who has not previously been diagnosed with diabetes has elevated blood glucose levels during pregnancy

glucagon-like peptide-1 (GLP-1): An incretin released from your intestine that makes you feel full after eating and slows the rate at which your stomach empties

glucagon-like peptide-1 (GLP-1) receptor agonists: An injectable class of type 2 diabetes medications that mimic the actions of GLP-1 (e.g., Victoza®)

glucose: Body fuel generated by your digestive system from the carbohydrates you eat, used by your cells for energy and stored in your liver and muscles

glycemic index (GI): A food ranking system that indicates how quickly foods containing carbohydrates get into your bloodstream

glycemic load (GL): A food ranking system that considers both glycemic index and portion size

glycogen: Extra glucose stored in your liver and muscles for future use

hemoglobin: Protein that distributes oxygen throughout your body

hemoglobin A1C (HbA1C): A blood test that indicates average blood glucose levels over the past three months

high-density lipoprotein (HDL): A "good" type of cholesterol that removes LDL cholesterol from the body

hormones: Chemicals secreted by the body to regulate processes like metabolism and reproduction

hyperglycemia: A state of high blood sugar which occurs when you don't have enough insulin to move glucose from your bloodstream to your cells

hypertension (high blood pressure): When the force of the blood pushing against the walls of your arteries is consistently too high

hypoglycemia: A state of low blood sugar, a life-threatening condition that occurs when you have too much insulin for the amount of glucose in your bloodstream

impaired fasting glucose (IFG): *See* impaired glucose tolerance

impaired glucose tolerance (IGT): Higher than normal blood glucose levels that are not high enough for a type 2 diabetes diagnosis, as measured by an oral glucose tolerance test. If you have IGT, your doctor will probably tell you that you have prediabetes.

incretins: Hormones in your gut that regulate the amount of insulin released after you eat

insoluble fiber: Fiber that does not digest at all and pushes food through your gastrointestinal tract

insulin: A hormone normally produced in the pancreas that regulates the amount of glucose in the blood, which must be injected by people with type 1 diabetes

insulin resistance (IR): A condition in which the body makes insulin but doesn't use it very effectively

irritable bowel syndrome (IBS): A condition affecting the large intestine that results in abdominal pain, bloating, and bowel system disturbances

lactose: A type of sugar found in milk products and some processed foods

latent autoimmune diabetes in adults (LADA): A type of diabetes with characteristics of both type 1 and type 2, sometimes called type 1.5

linoleic acid (LA): An omega-6 essential fatty acid

lipid: A type of fat in the blood, such as cholesterol and triglycerides

low-density lipoprotein (LDL): A "bad" type of cholesterol that collects in the walls of blood vessels and may cause blockages

lycopene: A substance in red foods like tomatoes that may help prevent heart disease and some cancers

macronutrients: Nutrients required by the body in large quantities, such as carbohydrates, protein, and fat

meglitinides: A class of type 2 diabetes medications that work like sulfonylureas but act much more quickly and may also cause hypoglycemia (e.g., Prandin®)

micronutrients: Nutrients required by the body in smaller quantities, like vitamins and minerals

monounsaturated fat: A type of fat found in foods like olive oil, avocado, and canola oil that lowers cholesterol and reduces your risk of heart disease and stroke

non-celiac wheat sensitivity: A condition in which someone is sensitive to the effects of wheat but doesn't test positive for celiac disease

omega-3 fatty acid: A type of fat found in fatty fish that may decrease risk of cardiovascular disease, combat insulin resistance, and lower triglycerides

omega-6 fatty acid: A type of fat found in nuts, seeds, and vegetable oils

plate method: A technique for estimating correct portion sizes

polycystic ovary syndrome (PCOS): A hormonal disorder in women of reproductive age characterized by metabolic problems, elevated levels of male hormones, menstrual cycle irregularities, and difficulty conceiving

polyunsaturated fat: A type of fat found in foods like corn oil, sunflower seeds, and walnuts that provides your body with essential fatty acids

portion size: The amount of a particular food you eat in one sitting

prediabetes: A condition where blood glucose is higher than normal, but not high enough for a diagnosis of type 2 diabetes

protein: A macronutrient found in foods like beef, pork, poultry, fish, eggs, cheese, beans, and soy that creates, maintains, and repairs tissues and cells in the body

registered dietitian (RD): A food and nutrition expert that has met certain academic and professional qualifications

saturated fat: A type of fat found in foods like fatty meat, poultry skin, and cream that raises cholesterol and increases your risk of heart disease and stroke

serving size: The amount of a particular food for which nutrition information has been calculated

sodium-glucose co-transporter 2 (SGLT2): A protein that tries to preserve the glucose your kidneys are attempting to eliminate from your body

sodium-glucose co-transporter 2 (SGLT2) inhibitors: A class of type 2 diabetes medications that block the effects of SGLT2, enabling the kidneys to eliminate glucose so as to lower blood sugar (e.g., Invokana®)

soluble fiber: Fiber that partially digests and remains gel-like to help remove cholesterol and toxins from your body

sucrose: A type of sugar that's a 50/50 blend of glucose and fructose (a.k.a. table sugar)

sugar alcohol: A type of sweetener containing carbs that digests slowly and has a minimal impact on blood sugar

sulfonylureas: A class of type 2 diabetes medications that stimulate the beta cells in the pancreas to release insulin and may cause hypoglycemia (e.g., glipizide)

thiazolidinediones: A class of type 2 diabetes medications that reduce insulin resistance and decrease the amount of glucose made by the liver (e.g., Avandia®)

trans fat: A type of fat found in processed foods that raises LDL cholesterol and lowers HDL cholesterol

triglycerides: A fat in the blood, too much of which may indicate insulin resistance and increase risk for coronary artery disease

type 1 diabetes: An autoimmune disorder in which the body attacks the beta cells in the pancreas responsible for making insulin

type 2 diabetes: A metabolic disorder characterized by high blood glucose and insulin resistance caused by both genetic and life-style factors

Resources

Carb-Counting and Tracking Websites, Apps, and Books

CalorieKing (calorieking.com), available in app, website, and book formats, provides nutritional information for numerous foods, including menu items from chain restaurants.

ControlMyWeight (calorieking.com/products/controlmyweight) is an app from the CalorieKing folks that offers meal and exercise tracking.

Lose It! (loseit.com) is an app and website that offers meal and exercise tracking.

MyFitnessPal (myfitnesspal.com) is another app and website providing meal and exercise tracking.

The Complete Book of Food Counts: The Book That Counts It All, by Corinne T. Netzer, is an indexed food database in book form only.

USDA Food Composition Databases (ndb.nal.usda.gov/ndb) is an online food database hub that serves as the engine for most carb-counting websites and apps.

Diabetes Information and Education

American Association of Diabetes Educators (diabeteseducator
.org) provides a search tool to help you find diabetes education
programs offered in your area.

American Diabetes Association (diabetes.org) is an organization
that provides programs, tools, and useful information to improve
the lives of people living with diabetes.

Create Your Plate (diabetes.org/food-and-fitness/food/planning
-meals/create-your-plate) is an interactive tool offered by the ADA
that explains the plate method.

Juvenile Diabetes Research Foundation (jdrf.org) is an organization that funds type 1 diabetes research.

The University of Sydney offers an entire website (glycemicindex
.com) on the glycemic index, including a search tool.

YMCA Diabetes Prevention Program (ymca.net
/diabetes-prevention) is available for people with prediabetes and
type 2 diabetes at many branches nationwide.

Diabetes Support

Diabetes Daily (diabetesdaily.com) offers information, articles, and
forums for people with diabetes.

Diabetes Mine (healthline.com/diabetesmine) is a "diabetes newspa-
per with a personal twist," written by and for people with diabetes.

DiabetesSisters (diabetessisters.org) is an organization offering education and peer support for adult women with any type of diabetes.

Diabetic Foodie (diabeticfoodie.com) is a website offering
diabetic-friendly recipes and tips for healthy eating.

diaTribe (diatribe.org) is a patient-focused online publication that
covers a wide variety of topics relating to diabetes.

dLife (dlife.com) offers Frequently Asked Questions (FAQs), recipes, and practical tips for people managing diabetes.

Taking Control of Your Diabetes (tcoyd.org) offers educational conferences for people with diabetes and accredited continuing medical education programs for health care providers.

TuDiabetes (tudiabetes.org) offers resources and forums in English and Spanish for both people with diabetes and their loved ones.

Fitness and Stress Management

Buddhify (buddhify.com) is an "on-the-go" app that offers meditations for specific situations (e.g., getting ready to sleep).

DiabetesStrong (diabetesstrong.com) offers exercise videos and other information important for people with diabetes who are physically active.

Headspace (headspace.com) is a meditation app featuring animations and videos.

NIDDK Body Weight Planner (niddk.nih.gov/health-information /weight-management/body-weight-planner) helps you figure out how many calories you need to consume each day based on your weight, sex, height, and activity level.

Finding Health Professionals

The National Certification Board for Diabetes Educators offers a tool (ncbde.org/find-a-cde/) to help you locate a **Certified Diabetes Educator (CDE)** in your area.

The Academy of Nutrition and Dietetics offers a tool (eatright.org /find-an-expert) to help you find a **Registered Dietitian (RD)** in your area.

References

American Diabetes Association. "About Our Meal Plans." Accessed January 17, 2018. www.diabetes.org/mfa-recipes /about-our-meal-plans.html

———— "Diagnosing Diabetes and Learning about Prediabetes." Last updated December 9, 2014. www.diabetes.org /are-you-at-risk/prediabetes/

———— "Standards of Medical Care in Diabetes—2018." *Diabetes Care*, 41 (Supplement 1). January 2018. care.diabetesjournals .org/content/diacare/suppl/2017/12/08/41.Supplement_1.DC1 /DC_41_S1_Combined.pdf

———— "Stress." Last updated December 6, 2013. www.diabetes .org/living-with-diabetes/complications/mental-health /stress.html

———— "Too Much or Too Little Sleep May Raise Your Blood Glucose Level and Expand Your Waistline." Last updated October 7, 2013. www.diabetes.org/research-and-practice /patient-access-to-research/too-much-or-too-little-sleep.html

American Heart Association. "Monounsaturated Fat." Last updated March 24, 2017. healthyforgood.heart.org/eat-smart /articles/monounsaturated-fats

————— "Polyunsaturated Fat." Last updated March 24, 2017. healthyforgood.heart.org/eat-smart/articles/polyunsaturated-fats

————— "Saturated Fat." Last updated March 24, 2017. healthyforgood.heart.org/eat-smart/articles/saturated-fats

————— "Trans Fat." Last updated March 24, 2017. healthyforgood.heart.org/eat-smart/articles/trans-fat

Blair, Elizabeth. "Insulin A to Z: A Guide on Different Types of Insulin." Joslin Diabetes Center. Accessed January 4, 2018. www.joslin.org/info/insulin_a_to_z_a_guide_on_different_types_of_insulin.html

Calentine, Leighann. "How the Food You Eat Affects Your Brain." *Diabetes Daily*. November 6, 2017. www.diabetesdaily.com/blog/how-the-food-you-eat-affects-your-brain-503081/

Campbell, Amy. "Diabetes Medicine: Alpha-Glucosidase Inhibitors." *Diabetes Self-Management*. August 31, 2015. www.diabetesselfmanagement.com/blog/diabetes-medicine-alpha-glucosidase-inhibitors/

————— "Diabetes Medicine: Bile Acid Sequestrants and Dopamine Receptor Agonists." *Diabetes Self-Management*. September 8, 2015. www.diabetesselfmanagement.com/blog/diabetes-medicine-bile-acid-sequestrants-and-dopamine-receptor-agonists/

————— "Diabetes Medicine: DPP-4 Inhibitors." *Diabetes Self-Management*. August 17, 2015. www.diabetesselfmanagement.com/blog/diabetes-medicine-dpp-4-inhibitors/

————— "Diabetes Medicine: Meglitinides." *Diabetes Self-Management*. August 3, 2015. www.diabetesselfmanagement.com/blog/diabetes-medicine-meglitinides/

———— "Diabetes Medicine: Metformin." *Diabetes Self-Management*. July 20, 2015. www.diabetesselfmanagement.com/blog/diabetes-medicine-metformin/

———— "Diabetes Medicine: SGLT2 Inhibitors." *Diabetes Self-Management*. August 24, 2015. www.diabetesselfmanagement.com/blog/diabetes-medicine-sglt2-inhibitors/

———— "Diabetes Medicine: Sulfonylureas." *Diabetes Self-Management*. July 27, 2015. www.diabetesselfmanagement.com/blog/diabetes-medicine-sulfonylureas/

———— "Diabetes Medicine: Thiazolidinediones." *Diabetes Self-Management*. August 10, 2015. www.diabetesselfmanagement.com/blog/diabetes-medicine-thiazolidinediones/

———— "Non-insulin Injectable Diabetes Medications." *Diabetes Self-Management*. September 14, 2015. www.diabetesselfmanagement.com/blog/non-insulin-injectable-diabetes-medications/

Celiac Disease Foundation. "What Is Celiac Disease?" Accessed January 15, 2018. celiac.org/celiac-disease/understanding-celiac-disease-2/what-is-celiac-disease/

Centers for Disease Control and Prevention (CDC). "Prediabetes." Last updated July 25, 2017. www.cdc.gov/diabetes/basics/prediabetes.html

Colberg, Sheri R., Ronald J. Sigal, Jane E. Yardley, Michael C. Riddell, David W. Dunstan, Paddy C. Dempsey, Edward S. Horton, Kristin Castorino, and Deborah F. Tate. "Physical Activity/Exercise and Diabetes: A Position Statement of the American Diabetes Association." *Diabetes Care*. November 2016. care.diabetesjournals.org/content/39/11/2065

Dandona, Paresh, and Ajay Chaudhuri. "Sodium-Glucose Co-Transporter 2 Inhibitors for Type 2 Diabetes Mellitus: An Overview for the Primary Care Physician." National Center for Biotechnology Information, April 24, 2017. www.ncbi .nlm.nih.gov/pmc/articles/PMC5518299/

Diabetes.co.uk. "Insulin Resistance." Accessed January 4, 2018. www.diabetes.co.uk/insulin-resistance.html

Dubois, Wil. "Ask D'Mine: Best Apps for Carb Counting?" *Diabetes Mine*. December 2, 2017. www.healthline.com /diabetesmine/ask-dmine-best-carb-counting-app

Evert, Alison B., Jackie L. Boucher, Marjorie Cypress, Stephanie A. Dunbar, Marion J. Franz, Elizabeth J. Mayer-Davis, Joshua J. Neumiller, Robin Nwankwo, Cassandra L. Verdi, Patti Urbanski, and William S. Yancy Jr. "Nutrition Therapy Recommendations for the Management of Adults with Diabetes." *Diabetes Care*. October 9, 2013. care.diabetesjournals.org /content/diacare/early/2013/10/07/dc13-2042.full.pdf

Gearing, Mary E. "Natural and Added Sugars: Two Sides of the Same Coin." Science in the News, Harvard University. Accessed January 15, 2018. sitn.hms.harvard.edu/flash/2015 /natural-and-added-sugars-two-sides-of-the-same-coin/

Hamdy, Osama, and Amy Campbell. "Diet and Diabetes: A Personalized Approach." Joslin Diabetes Center. November 25, 2005. www.joslin.org/info/diet_and_diabetes_a_personalized _approach.html

Harvard Health Publishing. "Glycemic Index for 60+ foods." Last updated March 14, 2018. www.health.harvard.edu/healthy -eating/glycemic-index-and-glycemic-load-for-100-foods

Harvard T. H. Chan School of Public Health. "Protein." Accessed January 15, 2018. www.hsph.harvard.edu/nutritionsource /what-should-you-eat/protein/

Health.gov. "Estimated Calorie Needs per Day, by Age, Sex, and Physical Activity Level." Accessed January 17, 2018. health .gov/dietaryguidelines/2015/guidelines/appendix-2/

Higdon, Jane. "Essential Fatty Acids." Oregon State University. Last updated May 2014. http://lpi.oregonstate.edu/mic/other -nutrients/essential-fatty-acids

Johns Hopkins Medicine. "Liver: Anatomy and Functions." Accessed January 4, 2018. www.hopkinsmedicine.org /healthlibrary/conditions/liver_biliary_and_pancreatic _disorders/liver_anatomy_and_functions_85,P00676

Johns Hopkins Patient Guide to Diabetes. "Sulfonylureas and Meglitinides." Accessed January 4, 2018. hopkinsdiabetesinfo.org/medications-for-type-2-diabetes-sulfo nylureas-and-meglitinides/

Johns Hopkins Patient Guide to Diabetes. "Thiazolidinediones." Accessed January 4, 2018. hopkinsdiabetesinfo.org /medications-for-type-2-diabetes-thiazolidinediones/

Kerns, Jennifer C., Juen Guo, Erin Fothergill, Lilian Howard, Nicolas D. Knuth, Robert Brychta, Kong Y. Chen, Monica C. Skarulis, Peter J. Walter, and Kevin D. Hall. "Increased Physical Activity Associated with Less Weight Regain Six Years after 'The Biggest Loser' Competition." *Obesity*. October 30, 2017. onlinelibrary.wiley.com/doi/10.1002/oby.21986/full

Leontis, Lisa M., and Amy Hess-Fischl. "Combination Medications for Type 2 Diabetes." EndocrineWeb. Last updated August 19, 2015. www.endocrineweb.com/conditions /type-2-diabetes/combination-medications-type-2-diabetes

Lewin, Jo. "Sugar Explained." BBC Good Food. Last updated July 28, 2017. www.bbcgoodfood.com/howto/guide/sugar -explained

MacMilian, Amanda, Jamie Ducharme, Markham Heid, and Alexandra Sifferlin. "8 Weight-Loss Strategies That Actually Work." *Time* 191, no. 4 (February 5, 2018): 50–53.

Mayo Clinic. "Acanthosis Nigricans." Accessed January 4, 2018. www.mayoclinic.org/diseases-conditions/acanthosis-nigricans /symptoms-causes/syc-20368983

——— "Hypoglycemia." Accessed January 4, 2018. www.mayoclinic .org/diseases-conditions/hypoglycemia/symptoms-causes /syc-20373685

——— "Insulin: Compare Common Options for Insulin Therapy." Accessed January 4, 2018. www.mayoclinic.org/diseases -conditions/diabetes/in-depth/insulin/art-20050970

——— "Nutrition and Healthy Eating." Accessed January 4, 2018. www.mayoclinic.org/healthy-lifestyle/nutrition-and -healthy-eating/in-depth/carbohydrates/art-20045705?p=1

——— "Type 2 Diabetes." Accessed January 4, 2018. www .mayoclinic.org/diseases-conditions/type-2-diabetes /diagnosis-treatment/drc-20351199

McKittrick, Martha, and Michelle Anderson. *The Type 2 Diabetic Cookbook and Action Plan*. Berkeley: Rockridge Press, 2017.

National Academy of Sciences. "Dietary Reference Intakes for Energy, Carbohydrate, Fiber, Fat, Fatty Acids, Cholesterol, Protein, and Amino Acids." September 5, 2002. www .nationalacademies.org/hmd/Reports/2002/Dietary-Reference -Intakes-for-Energy-Carbohydrate-Fiber-Fat-Fatty-Acids -Cholesterol-Protein-and-Amino-Acids.aspx

National Institute of Diabetes and Digestive and Kidney Diseases (NIDDK). "Diabetes, Heart Disease, and Stroke." Last updated February 2017. www.niddk.nih.gov/health-information /diabetes/overview/preventing-problems/heart-disease-stroke

——— "Low Blood Glucose (Hypoglycemia)." Last updated August 2016. www.niddk.nih.gov/health-information /diabetes/overview/preventing-problems/low-blood-glucose -hypoglycemia

——— "Your Digestive System & How It Works." Accessed January 4, 2018. www.niddk.nih.gov/health-information /digestive-diseases/digestive-system-how-it-works

National Institutes of Health (NIH). "Omega-3 Fatty Acids." Last updated November 2, 2016. ods.od.nih.gov/factsheets /Omega3FattyAcids-HealthProfessional/

National Sleep Foundation. "How Much Sleep Do We Really Need?" Accessed February 2, 2018. sleepfoundation.org /excessivesleepiness/content/how-much-sleep-do-we-really -need-0

Pallant, Ben, and Payal Marathe. "FDA Approves Ozempic, a Powerful Once-Weekly Type 2 Diabetes Medication." *diaTribe*. December 11, 2017. diatribe.org/fda-approves -ozempic-powerful-once-weekly-type-2-diabetes-medication

Pasquale, Di. "The Essentials of Essential Fatty Acids." PubMed. Accessed January 15, 2018. www.ncbi.nlm.nih.gov /pubmed/22435414

Prasad-Reddy, Lalita, and Diana Isaacs. "A Clinical Review of GLP-1 Receptor Agonists: Efficacy and Safety in Diabetes and Beyond." National Center for Biotechnology Information. July 9, 2015. www.ncbi.nlm.nih.gov/pmc/articles/PMC4509428/

PubMed Health. "Gastrointestinal Tract (GI Tract)." Accessed January 4, 2018. www.ncbi.nlm.nih.gov/pubmedhealth /PMHT0022855/

Rodibaugh, Rosemary. "The Exchange List System for Diabetic Meal Planning." University of Arkansas Division of Agriculture Cooperative Extension Service. Accessed January 19, 2018. www.uaex.edu/publications/pdf/FSHED-86.pdf

Scheiner, Gary. *The Ultimate Guide to Accurate Carb Counting.* Cambridge, MA: Da Capo Press, 2006.

SELF NutritionData. "Glycemic Index." Accessed February 2, 2018. nutritiondata.self.com/topics/glycemic-index

Shafer, Sherri. *Diabetes & Carb Counting for Dummies.* Hoboken: John Wiley & Sons, Inc., 2017.

Sola, Daniele, Luca Rossi, Gian Piero Carnevale Schianca, Pamela Maffioli, Marcello Bigliocca, Robert Mella, Francesca Corliano, Gian Paolo Fra, Ettore Bartoli, and Giuseppe Derosa. "Sulfonylureas and Their Use in Clinical Practice." National Center for Biotechnology Information. August 11, 2015. www.ncbi.nlm.nih.gov/pmc/articles/PMC4548036/

Spritzler, Franziska. "How Many Carbs Should a Diabetic Eat?" Healthline. Accessed January 17, 2018. www.healthline.com /nutrition/diabetes-carbs-per-day#section3

Strawbridge, Holly. "Artificial Sweeteners: Sugar-free, but at What Cost?" Harvard Health (blog). July 16, 2012. www.health.harvard.edu/blog/artificial-sweeteners-sugar -free-but-at-what-cost-201207165030

Thomas, Clayton L., ed., *Taber's Cyclopedic Medical Dictionary*, 18th edition. Philadelphia: F.A. Davis Company, 1993.

Tsai, Allison, and Erin Palinski-Wade. "Debunking Claims about Advanced Carb Counting." *Diabetes Forecast*. July 2017. Accessed February 2, 2018. www.diabetesforecast.org/2017 /jul-aug/debunking-claims-about.html

University of California San Francisco SugarScience. "Hidden in Plain Sight." Accessed January 4, 2018. sugarscience.ucsf.edu /hidden-in-plain-sight/#.Wk_w9NuZO9Y

———— "How Much is Too Much? The Growing Concern over Too Much Added Sugar in Our Diets." Accessed January 30, 2018. sugarscience.ucsf.edu/the-growing-concern-of -overconsumption

U.S. Department of Agriculture (USDA) National Agricultural Library. "Macronutrients." Accessed January 4, 2018. www.nal.usda.gov/fnic/macronutrients

U.S. Food and Drug Administration (FDA). "Additional Information about High-Intensity Sweeteners Permitted for Use in Food in the United States." Last updated February 8, 2018. www.fda.gov/food/ingredientspackaginglabeling /foodadditivesingredients/ucm397725.htm

———— "Changes to the Nutrition Facts Label." Last updated March 15, 2018. https://www.fda.gov/food/guidanceregulation /guidancedocumentsregulatoryinformation/labelingnutrition /ucm385663.htm

———— "Dietary Fiber." Accessed January 4, 2018. www. accessdata.fda.gov/scripts/InteractiveNutritionFactsLabel /dietary-fiber.html

———— "FDA-Approved Diabetes Medications." Last updated February 2, 2018. www.fda.gov/ForPatients/Illness/Diabetes /ucm408682.htm

———— "FDA Drug Safety Communication: FDA Requires Removal of Some Prescribing and Dispensing Restrictions for Rosiglitazone-Containing Diabetes Medications." Last updated August 1, 2017. www.fda.gov/Drugs/DrugSafety/ucm376389.htm

———— "FDA Drug Safety Communication: FDA Warns That DPP-4 Inhibitors for Type 2 Diabetes May Cause Severe Joint Pain." Last updated August 28, 2015. www.fda.gov/Drugs/DrugSafety/ucm459579.htm

U.S. National Library of Medicine Medline Plus. "Carbohydrates." Accessed January 4, 2018. medlineplus.gov/carbohydrates.html

———— "Dietary Proteins." Accessed January 15, 2018. medlineplus.gov/dietaryproteins.html

Warshaw, Hope S., and Karmeen Kulkarni. *Complete Guide to Carb Counting*, 2nd edition. American Diabetes Association, 2004.

Youdim, Adrienne. "Carbohydrates, Proteins, and Fats." Merck Manual Consumer Version. Accessed January 4, 2018. www.merckmanuals.com/home/disorders-of-nutrition/overview-of-nutrition/carbohydrates,-proteins,-and-fats

Index

About the Author

Shelby Kinnaird publishes diabetic-friendly recipes and tips on healthy eating at Diabetic Foodie (www.diabeticfoodie.com), a website often stamped with a "top diabetes blog" label. She loves food, hence her motto: "A diabetes diagnosis is not a dietary death sentence." A passionate diabetes advocate, Shelby likes to make her voice heard and writes for websites like *Healthline* and the DiabetesSisters blog. She leads two diabetes support groups in the Richmond, Virginia, area and has successfully managed her type 2 diabetes since 1999.

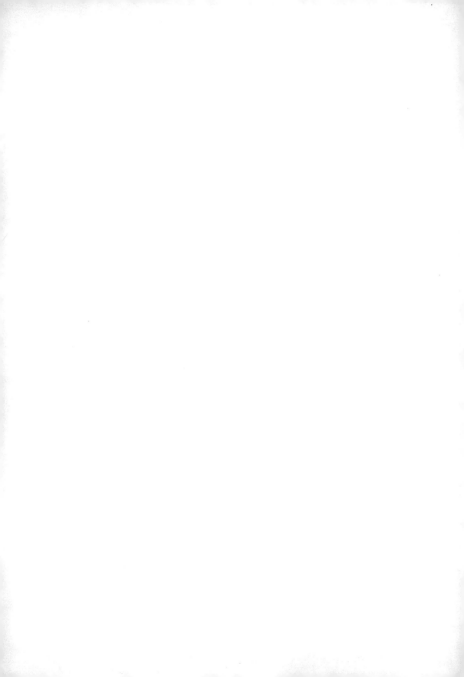

CPSIA information can be obtained
at www.ICGtesting.com
Printed in the USA
JSHW032309241121
20738JS00004B/6

9 781641 520652